*Each page of this book
has stolen hours from our family life.
We hope that our Wives Layla and Brunella
will appreciate this repairing dedication*

Springer
Berlin
Heidelberg
New York
Barcelona
Budapest
Hong Kong
London
Milano
Paris
Tokyo

Luigi Allegra - Francesco Blasi (Eds.)

Chlamydia Pneumoniae Infection

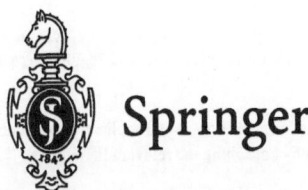

Springer

Prof. Luigi Allegra, M.D.
Head of the Institute of Respiratory Diseases
University of Milan
Via Francesco Sforza 35 - Milan
Italy

Dr. Francesco Blasi, M.D., PH.D.
Assistant Professor, Institute of Respiratory Diseases
University of Milan
Via Francesco Sforza 35 - Milan
Italy

ISBN-13:978-3-540-75007-9   e-ISBN-13: 978-88-470-2201-0
DOI: 10.1007/978-88-470-2201-0

Table of Contents

Contributors

LUIGI ALLEGRA, M.D.
Full Professor, Head of the Institute of Respiratory Diseases,
University of Milan, Italy

FRANCESCO BLASI, M.D., PH.D.
Assistant Professor, Institute of Respiratory Diseases,
University of Milan, Italy

ROBERTO COSENTINI, M.D.
First Assistant, Emergency Medicine Department,
Ospedale Maggiore, Milan, Italy

BENJAMIN DAVIES, M.D., FRC Path.
Director, Medical Microbiology,
De Wever Ziekenhuis, Heerlen, The Nederlands

FRANCO DENTI, M.D.
First Assistant, Institute of Respiratory Diseases,
University of Milan, Italy

GIULIANA GIALDRONI GRASSI, M.D.
Full Professor, Institute of Chemotherapy,
University of Pavia, Italy

DAVID L. HAHN, M.D.
Arcand Park Clinic,
Madison, WI, USA

KIRSI LAITINEN, PH.D.
Laboratory for Respiratory Bacterial Infections,
NPHI, Oulu, Finland

AINO LAURILA, M.D., PH.D.
Laboratory for Respiratory Bacterial Infections,
NPHI, Oulu, Finland

MAIJA LEINONEN, PH.D.
Research Professor, Laboratory for Respiratory Bacterial Infections
NPHI, Oulu, Finland

FRANCIS P.V. MAESEN, M.D., FCCP
Director, Department of Respiratory Diseases,
De Wever Ziekenhuis, Heerlen, The Nederlands

JEANNE ORFILA, M.D.
Director, Laboratoire de Bacteriologie-Immunologie Generale,
Amiens, France

PEKKA SAIKKU, M.D.
Research Professor, Chlamydia Laboratory,
NPHI, Oulu, Finland

HELJÄ-MARIA SURCEL, PH.D.
Laboratory for Respiratory Bacterial Infections,
NPHI, Oulu, Finland

PAOLO TARSIA, M.D.
Fellow, Institute of Respiratory Diseases,
University of Milan, Italy

Chapter 1   History of a New Agent of Pneumonia

Luigi Allegra

The recognition of *Chlamydia pneumoniae* as a separate species within the *Chlamydia* genus is relatively recent [1], but clues in literature for the existence of this agent date back to at least 50 years ago. In the paper *Atypical pneumonia and psittacosis* published on the *Journal of Clinical Investigation* in 1943 [2], Smadel described cases of pneumonia with a positive complement fixation test for psittacosis but no history of past contact with birds. The Author concluded that "it appears desirable to search for a humanized strain (...) which is moderately contagious for man and which is transmitted from man to man by way of the upper respiratory route". Smadel's intuition remained "vox clamantis in deserto".

A second piece of the puzzle was put in place in 1965. During a trachoma vaccine trial performed in Taiwan, an atypical strain of *Chlamydia* obtained from the conjunctiva of a primary school control child, was identified on the yolk sac chick embryo egg number 183. The strain was therefore named TW-183 (TW = Taiwan).

A further step was made in 1983 when another isolate antigenically similar to TW-183 was obtained from the pharyngeal swab of a Washington University student in Seattle affected by pharyngitis and the strain was named AR-39 (AR = acute respiratory).

Between 1985 and 1986 two studies were published on the clinical relevance of respiratory infections sustained by an unusual strain of *Chlamydia psittaci* [3, 4]. Saikku in 1985 reported an epidemic of mild pneumonia discovered during a chest radiographic survey of young adults in two communities in Finland. The following year Grayston described a series of isolations of a *Chlamydia psittaci* strain within a population of university students with respiratory tract infections. The Authors named the strain TWAR, from the designation of the first two isolates, TW-183 and AR-39. Following ultrastructural definition and DNA homology analysis the puzzle was finally completed in 1989 with the classification of a third species of *Chlamydia* named *Chlamydia pneumoniae* sp. nov. [1].

Since 1989 a growing number of reports indicating *Chlamydia pneumoniae* as a common cause of lower respiratory infections have appeared worldwide, and it is now known that the seroprevalence for this agent is high, ranging between 40 and 70% in the adult population [5, 6]. It has also been suggested that *Chlamydia pneumoniae* infection may play a role in a multifactorial disease such as bronchial asthma [7, 8]. Furthermore, this agent has recently been held responsable for acute non respiratory diseases such as myocarditis, endocarditis and erythema nodosum [9, 10]. Starting from 1988 Saikku has been exploring the possibility of a correlation between chronic infection with *Chlamydia pneumoniae* and coronary artery disease [11, 12].

Given the clinical and epidemiological importance of this micro-organism we feel an updated focus on the different aspects of *Chlamydia pneumoniae* infection will be a useful *vademecum* for both physicians and scientists involved in this ever changing field. The presence amongst the Authors of one of the fathers of *Chlamydia pneumoniae* allows us to be confident that the end result will have been worth our efforts and will fulfill our hopes.

References

1. Grayston JT, Kuo CC, Campbell LA, Wang SP (1989) *Chlamydia pneumoniae* sp. nov. for Chlamydia sp strain TWAR. Int J Syst Bacteriol 39:88-90
2. Smadel JE (1943) Atypical pneumonia and psittacosis. J Clin Invest 22:57-65
3. Saikku P, Wang SP, Kleemola M, Brander E et al (1985) An epidemic of mild pneumonia due to an unusual strain of *Chlamydia psittaci*. J Infect Dis 151:832-839
4. Grayston JT, Kuo CC, Wang SP, Altman T (1986) A new *Chlamydia psittaci*, strain TWAR, isolated in acute respiratory tract infections. N Engl J Med 315:161-168
5. Grayston JT, Campbell LA, Kuo CC et al (1990) A new respiratory tract pathogen: *Chlamydia pneumoniae* strain TWAR. J Infect Dis 161:618-625
6. Marrie TJ (1993) *Chlamydia pneumoniae*. Thorax 48:1-4
7. Hahn DL, Dodge RW, Golubjatnikov R (1991) Association of *Chlamydia pneumoniae* (strain TWAR) infection with wheezing, asthmatic bronchitis, and adult-onset asthma. JAMA 266:225-230
8. Allegra L, Blasi F, Centanni S, Cosentini R, Denti F, Raccanelli R et al (1994) Acute exacerbations of asthma in adults: role of *Chlamydia pneumoniae* infection. Eur Respir J 7:2165-2168
9. Marrie TJ, Harczy M, Mann OE, Landymore RW, Raza A, Wang SP, Grayston JT (1990) Culture negative endocarditis probably due to *Chlamydia pneumoniae*. J Infect Dis 161:127-129
10. Persson K (1990) Epidemiological and clinical aspects on infections due to *Chlamydia pneumoniae* (strain TWAR). Scand J Infect Dis S69:63-67
11. Saikku P, Leinonen M, Mattila K, Ekman MR, Nieminen MS, Makela PH et al (1988) Serological evidence of an association of a novel *Chlamydia* TWAR, with chronic coronary artery disease and acute myocardial infarction. Lancet ii:983-986
12. Saikku P, Leinonen M, Tenkanen L, Linnanmaki E, Ekman MR, Manninen V et al (1992) Chronic *Chlamydia pneumoniae* infection as a risk factor for coronary heart disease in the Helsinki Heart Study. Ann Intern Med 116:273-278

Chapter 2   *Chlamydia pneumoniae* Microbiology

Jeanne Orfila

Introduction

The discovery of a new micro-organism is an exciting experience for the microbiologist. Once a hard work, it is now made easier by the new techniques. This is what happened for *Chlamydia pneumoniae*.

Taxonomy

The Chlamydia genus comprises the bacteria that grow inside intracytoplasmic vacuoles by means of a complex cycle. They are Gram negative organisms with a reduced metabolism.

Chlamydiaceae are a single family including only the genus *Chlamydia*. The antigenic structure, the characteristics of multiplication and the DNA composition allow the differentiation of three species:

Chlamydia psittaci, found in several animal species, specially birds and mammalians, is the causative agent of lung diseases and abortion. However, it is frequently present in a quiescent form, giving rise to possible reactivation. Humans are infected by contact with animals and develop an atypical pneumonia with various degrees of severity, and possible cardiac, hepatic and central nervous involvement. An infective abortion might also occur in pregnant women.

Chlamydia trachomatis infection occurs almost exclusively in humans. It is responsable of trachoma, a serious ocular disease, and sexually transmitted infections, possibly leading to sterility.

Chlamydia pneumoniae is a primary human pathogen, where it generally causes respiratory tract infections as pharyngitis, bronchitis and atypical pneumonia. The infection is transmitted from human to human by the respiratory route, thus explaining the high prevalence of this pathogen in the general population [2, 3].

Cycle of replication

The modality of replication is a characteristic of the genus of *Chlamydia*, and the three species show the same complex cycle.

The cycle of replication has been studied after cell culture inoculation by means of optic and electron microscopy. *C. psittaci* and *C. trachomatis* have been evaluated extensively, whereas few reports refer to *C. pneumoniae*.

Photon Microscopy [4]

The specimens obtained few hours after inoculation and stained with giemsa do not yet show any intracellular modification. Only 10 to 12 hours after infection a small, round, dark blue mass becomes visible, often swelled, and blackberry-shaped (from that the name *morula*). It is particularly dense and limited in the species *C. pneumoniae*. After 20 to 24 hours the morula grows in size, and loses in part its homogeneity. It is visible inside several bluish granules. At 48th hour the inclusion of *C. pneumoniae* grows rapidly and, in contrast to the other species, where several granules of different colour and size appear, the greatest ones rest bluish, and the smallest change to dark purple, the inclusion of *C. pneumoniae* remains round and dense, growing slowly and entering a part of the cytoplasm.

Sometimes several inclusions are found inside the same cell, like a pearl string around the nucleus. This aspect is typical of *C. pneumoniae*, suggesting that fusion of inclusion does not occur, in contrast to the species of *C. trachomatis*. This characteristic approaches *C. pneumoniae* to *C. psittaci*; some inclusions appearing in the same cell of morula are very large, pointing out the possibility of a second cycle of replication in the same cell. Ninetytwo hours after infection the host cell blows up and several particules are released in the medium.

The techniques of photon microscopy do not allow the observation of the inclusions during the first hours following cell inoculation. The first Authors hypothesized a sort of eclipse, but electron microscopy confuted this speculation. However, the contrast phase microscopy, turning in microcinema, showed that the host cells remain in good health for a long time, since they can still divide. Each of the derived cell retains a fragment of the inclusion that subsequently divides and develops normally.

Electron Microscopy [5]

With the study of electron microscopy the hypotesis of eclipse, the disappearance of the micro-organism, proved to be false. The infective particle enters inside the cell and some minutes to hours after inoculation a small particle, 0.3 um diameter, with a paracentral nucleulus, a zone with granulations, and a well defined wall are found [6]. This particle, called elementary body (EB), is found inside a vacuole of phagocytosis. Whereas all Authors agree about the spheric shape of *C. psittaci* and *C. trachomatis* elementary bodies, the ultrastructure of *C. pneumoniae* elementary bodies is still debated. In fact, Campbell, Kuo and Grayston [7] showed that elementary bodies from isolate TWAR 183 cultured in HeLa cells seemed pear-shaped at electron microscopy. This characteristic allowed the differentiation from the other two species. For these Authors the elementary bodies appeared pleiomorphic with a predominance of a piriform shape, showing a round cytoplasmatic mass and a large periplasmic space. For these Authors the sharp point of the EB might play a role in the bacterial adhesion to the host cell. They propose to consider this characteristic in order to define species. However, other Authors working on different isolates, i.e. Carter [8] on IOL 207 and ATCC VR 1310, Kanamoto on YK 41 [9], Popov on IOL [10], observed perfectly round elementary bodies identical to those seen in *C. trachomatis* and *C. psittaci*. To our opinion the morphology of EBs is still an open dilemma and should not be considered among classification criteria.

The EB, inside the vacuole of phagocytosis, grows progressively in diameter until 0.6 to 1 um, and is surrounded by a thin wall; the inner part of the cytoplasm is homogeneous, without a nucleus. These elements, called reticulate bodies (RBs), are always grouped in a vacuole that is growing according to multiplication, as seen in other species, with inhibition of lysosome-phagosome fusion. There are images of binary division, and the number of reticulates bodies increases. The structure of RBs is identical in the different species. Electron microscopy shows that the *morula* observed on photon microscopy is composed by the agglomeration of RBs, with some of them about to divide. After some hours the inclusion will be formed only by RBs that undergo a modification of the morphology leading to the transformation, first into intermediate bodies by central DNA condensation, and finally to EBs. At this point the inclusion consists of three kinds of particulates: reticulate, intermediate, and elementary bodies. As the inclusion grows, the number of EBs increases, yet some reticulate bodies persist, usually at the border of the inclusion.

In conclusion, the electron microscopy showed three important findings: the characteristical structure of the microorganism, the lack of the eclipse phenomenon, and the existence of a complex cycle. During this cycle, the EB (infective particle) enters the host cell by phagocytosis, and subsequently changes into reticulate body, which represents the vegetative form of the organism, the only one capable of binary division. Then, the reticulate bodies generate the intermediate bodies which change into smaller EBs with a thicker wall. The release of these different particles allow the EBs to infect another cell [11]. Carter studied the three species concurrently and reported the presence of mini cells inside the inclusion and the relative paucity of EBs. This finding could explain the weak infectivity of *C. pneumoniae* in culture. Finally, we report that neither photon nor electron microscopy revealed the presence of glycogen. This characteristic differentiates *C. pneumoniae* from *C. trachomatis* and approaches *C. pneumoniae* to *C. psittaci*.

Antigenic Characteristics

The study of antigenic structure of *C. pneumoniae* has taken advantage from the data about *C. trachomatis* and *C. psittaci*. They demonstrated the existence in these two species of specific antigens allowing the subdivision of *Chlamydiaceae* family into genus, species, and serovars.

Genus Antigens

The demonstration of a lipopolysaccharidic genus antigen was performed by fluoresceinated monoclonal antibodies against the LPS of the two well known species. When this procedure was applied to *C. pneumoniae* the presence of this antigen was shown by the coloration of the inclusion in a homogeneous fashion. The LPS is present in the EBs and reticulate bodies outer membrane. It is composed by fatty acid and phospholipides [12]. The immunodominant determinant is a 2-ceto-desoxyoctanoic acid. The LPS presents at least two epitopes. One is shared with enterobacteria, the other one is specific to *Chlamydia* genus [13]. However, the LPS is not completely identical among the three species of *Chlamydia*. The *C. trachomatis* and *C. psittaci* glycoryl-transferase do not present an identical chemical structure and seem to be species-specific [14].

The LPS is thermostable. It is extracted by heating at 60° for 30 minutes with ether, acid, alcalis, and desoxycholate. It is inactivated by periodate. The lipid portion A of LPS presents three epitopes similar to those localised on LPS in other bacteria [15].

The composition of *C. pneumoniae* LPS in terms of fatty acids is very similar to *C. trachomatis* and *C. psittaci*, but is different for the presence of long chain acids (C22, C24, C26).

LPS is detectable about 30 hours after infection, in concurrence with inclusion maturation. It is present throughout the cycle, may enter the host cell, be incorporated in the cell membrane and released in the culture medium.

During *Chlamydia* infection the anti-genus antibodies (Abs) appear only with deep infection. In the course of the primary *C. pneumoniae* infection the anti-genus antibodies appear the first in an early phase.

Species Antigens

The differentiation of species antigens (Ag) and serovars is performed by the utilisation of the microimmunofluorescence (MIF) technique studied by Wang for *C. trachomatis*. This differentiation occurs with the use of polyclonal Abs from mice or, preferably, by monoclonal Abs [16].

The determinant of species antigens is the major outer membrane protein (MOMP) which is present in both EBs and reticulate bodies. In *C. trachomatis*, where it has been extensively studied, it represents 60% of outer membrane proteins. Its molecular weight varies according to the species from 39 to 45 kD for *C. trachomatis*, 38 to 40 kD for *C. psittaci*, from 39.5 kD for *C. pneumoniae* [17].

It contains four variable domains. The cartography of epitopes carried out for *C. trachomatis* showed that three domains, I, II, IV, present the specific antigenic determinants of serovars and sub-species. The domain IV is found on the C-terminal extremity of the protein and represents the determinant of the species [18,19].

The epitopes responsible for the species-specificity are found on the surface of the micro-organism and present a strong immunogenic power. They induce the appearance of neutralising Abs, an important step in the pathogenicity of the bacterium. However, they are sensitive to SDS denaturation, as demonstrated by Christiansen at al. [18] suggesting a tertiary or quaternary structure. Immunoblot analysis should consider this finding because *C. pneumoniae* immunogenicity be labelled weak compared to *C. trachomatis* and *C. psittaci*.

During *C. trachomatis* infection only the anti-species Abs appear. In contrast, during primary *C. pneumoniae* infection they appear late after anti-LPS Abs.

Type Antigens

Wang et al. [20] discovered these Ags in 1974 by MIF technique. Since 1960, in fact, the utilisation of a "test for the prevention of toxicity in mice" had allowed the definition of some serovars of *C. trachomatis*. Concordant results were obtained with MIF [20]. These thermolable Ags are found on the MOMP.

To date, at least 18 *C. trachomatis* serovars have been identified. *C. psittaci* serovars are numerous, and only thirteen have been classified. There are some differences between avian and mammalian isolates. The differentiation of the various serovars of *C. trachomatis* depends on the variation of the genus coding for the MOMP. The structure of *C. pneumoniae* MOMP is identical to that of *C. trachomatis* and variations of the encoding gene have not yet been found [21].

Several studies addressed the question of the number of serovars, but the evaluation of the specific antigens is hampered by the difficulty of *C. pneumoniae* culture and the rarity of the isolates. With the aid of the MIF technique, Wang studied 8 different isolates of *C. pneumoniae* from various countries. All reacted in the same way with both the serum of the corresponding patient and the specific monoclonal of every serovar. Moreover, Kanamoto found identical the peptidic profile of three different isolates of *C. pneumoniae*, TW 183, YK 41 and AR 39.

However, the work of Black with immunoelectrophoresis and 16 SrDNA study on isolates from USA and Norway suggest the existence of three serovars [22, 23]. Two would be human with two genotypes, the third would be equine [24].

Further studies are needed in order to improve the knowledge of antigen variation of *C. pneumoniae* species. To date, no reliable epidemiologic markers are available.

Antigens of the Group of the Heat-Shock Protein (HSP)

The group of the HSP represents a family of proteins involved in the elaboration of proteins from their synthesis to the assembly of multinumeric complexes. They are found in both eukaryotes and prokariotes [25].

A 57 kD HSP has been found in a proteic fraction of *C. trachomatis* inducing a late hypersensitivity reaction in the eyes of an India pig or a monkey sensitized with a prior *Chlamydia* infection. This protein is a genus-specific Ag and is similar to the protein GrEL in E. Coli (FK). The HSP57 is the second protein in terms of concentration in the lysates of *Chlamydia*. It is weakly bound to the cell surface and is present in EBs and RBs. It is present in all serovars of *C. trachomatis*. There is a great homology between the sequence of *Chlamydias'* HSP57 and human HSP60.

The HSP57 presents 13 major epitopes that are recognized by human sera. Seven out of 13 present a cross reaction with the human HSP60. These epitopes are species- and genus-specific and are thus shared by the three species. Another 75 kD HSP is synthetised early during the development cycle. This protein is cytoplasmic and is recognized by human sera on immunoblotting. It presents a 57% homology with E.Coli DNAK proteins, and 42% homology with human HSP60. In eukariotic cells, HSP70 are involved in the protein translocation through the cytoplasmic membrane and the unfolding of the protein secondary structure. The role of DNAK-like proteins in the *Chlamydias* has not been yet clarified. Anti-HSP75 antibodies recognize the EB's and neutralize the infection in vitro. The *C. pneumoniae* HSP75 share 87% homology with *C. trachomatis* HSP75 [26].

Few questions remain on the role of *C. pneumoniae* HSP in the physiopathology of infection. Is there a species-specific or an infection by one species sensitized against the others? Will be possible to identify a marker of severity of *C. pneumoniae* infection, specially in cardiac involvement, as in case of *C. trachomatis*? [27].

In conclusion, we would like to point out the difficulty of the study of immune response due to the similarity of the three species and the complexity of the structure.

References

1. Grayston JT, Kuo CC, Campbell LA, Wang SP (1989) *Chlamydia pneumoniae* sp nov. for Chlamydia sp strain TWAR. Intern J Syst Bacteriol 39:88-90
2. Grayston JT, Kuo CC, Wang SP, Altman DJ (1986) A new *Chlamydia psittaci* strain TWAR isolated in acute respiratory tract infections. N Engl J Med 315:161-168
3. Grayston JT, Wang SP, Kuo CC, Campbell LA (1989) Current knowledge on *Chlamydia pneumoniae* strain TWAR: an important cause of pneumonia and other acute respiratory diseases. Eur J Clin Microbiol Inf Dis 8:191-202
4. Lepinay A, Robineaux R, Orfila J, Moncel C, Coet H, Boutry JM (1971) Analyse en microcinématographie à contraste de phase du développement intracellulaire de *Chlamydia psittaci*. Archiv Fur die gesamte virusforschung 35:161-176
5. Lepinay A, Orfila J, Anteunis A, Boutry JM, Orme-Rosselli L, Robineaux R (1970) Etude en microscopie électronique du développement et de la morphologie de l'agent de l'Ornithose dans les macrophages de souris. Ann Inst Pasteur 119:222-231
6. Zhang JP, Stephens RS (1992) Mechanism of *Chlamydia trachomatis* attachment to eukarytic host cell. Cell 69:861-869
7. Campbell LA, Kuo CC, Grayston JT (1987) Characterisation of the new *Chlamydia* agent, TWAR, as a unique organism by restriction endonuclease analysis and DNA-DNA hybridization. J Clin Microbiol 25:1911-1916
8. Carter MW, Mahadawi AL, Giles IG, Treharne JD, Ward ME, Clarke IN (1991) Nucleotide sequence and taxonomic value of the major outer membrane protein gene of *Chlamydia pneumoniae* IOL 207. J Gen Microbiol 137:465-475
9. Kanamoto Y, Jijima Y, Miyashita N, Matsumoto A, Sanako T (1993) Antigenic characterisation of *Chlamydia pneumoniae* isolated in Hiroshima Japan. Microbiol Immunol 37:495-498
10. Popov VL, Shatkin AA, Pankratova VN, Smirnova NS et al (1991) Ultrastructure of

Chlamydia pneumoniae in cell culture. FEMS Microbiol Lett 84:129-134

11. Moulder JW (1991) Interaction of *Chlamydiae* and host cell in vitro. Microbiol Rev 55:143-190

12. Brade H, Baumann M, Brade L, Fu Y et al (1992) Chlamydial LPS structure and antigenic properties. In: Mardh PA, La Placa M, Ward M (eds) Second proceeding of the European Society for Chlamydia research. Società Editrice Esculapio, Bologna, Italy, pp 10-13

13. Nurminen M, Leinonen M, Saikku P, Makela PH (1983) The genus specific antigen of *Chlamydia* resemblance to the lipopolysaccharide of enteric bacteria. Science 220:1279-1281

14. Mamat U, Baumann M, Schmidt G, Brade H (1993) The genus specific lipopolysaccharide epiope of *Chlamydia* is assembled in *Chlamydia psittaci* and *Chlamydia trachomatis* by glycotransferase of low homology. Molecular Microbiol 10:935-941

15. Schrame KS, Kazar S, Sadecky E (1980) Serological cross reaction of lipid A components of LPS isolated from *Chlamydia psittaci* and *Coxiella burneti*. Acta virologica 24:224-230

16. Poulakkinen M, Parker J, Kuo CC, Grayston JT, Campbell LA (1994) Characterization of a *Chlamydia pneumoniae* epitope recognized by species specific monoclonal antibodies. Proceedings of the Eighth International Symposium on Human Chlamydial Infections. Orfila J et al (eds) Società Editrice Esculapio, Bologna, Italy, pp 185-188

17. Campbell LA, Kuo CC, Grayston JT (1990) Structural and antigenic analysis of *Chlamydia pneumoniae*. Inf Immun 58:93-97

18. Christansen L, Ostergaard L, Birkelund S (1994) Analysis of the *Chlamydia pneumoniae* surface. Proceedings of the Eighth International Symposium on Human Chlamydial Infections. Orfila J et al (eds) Società Editrice Esculapio Bologna, Italy, pp 173-177

19. Gaydos CA, Quinn TC, Bobo La, Eiden JJ (1992) Similarity of *Chlamydia pneumoniae* strains in the variable domain IV region of the major outer membrane protein gene. Inf Immun 60:5319-5323

20. Wang SP, Grayston JT (1994) The similarity of *Chlamydia pneumoniae* isolates as antigen in the microimmunofluorescence test. Proceedings of the Eighth International Symposium on Human Chlamydial Infections. Orfila J et al (eds) Società Editrice Esculapio, Bologna, Italy pp 181-184

21. Kornak JM, Kuo CC, Campbell LA (1991) Sequence analysis of the gene encoding the *Chlamydia pneumoniae* DNA k protein homolog. Infect Immun 59:721-725

22. Black CN, Petterson B, Messmer TO, Storey C, Uhlen M, Olsvik O (1994) Identification of three types of 16SrDNA genes in *Chlamydia pneumoniae* strains of human and non human origin. Proceedings of the Eighth International Symposium on Human Chlamydial Infections. Orfila J et al (eds) Società Editrice Esculapio, Bologna, Italy, pp 193-196

23. Black CN, Johnson JE, Farshy CE, Brown TM, Berdal BP (1991) Antigenic variation among strains of *Chlamydia pneumoniae*. J Clin Microbiol 29:1312-1316

24. Storey C, Lusher M, Yates P, Richmond S (1993) Evidence for *Chlamydia pneumoniae* of non human origin. J Gen Microbiol 139:2621-2626

25. Danilition SL, Maclean IW, Peeling R, Winston S, Brunham RC (1990) The 75-Kilodalton protein of *Chlamydia trachomatis*: a member of the heat shock protein 70 family? Inf Immun 58:189-196

26. Peeling RW, Toye B, Claman P, Jessamine P, Laferierre C (1994) Seropositivity to *Chlamydia pneumoniae* and antibody response to the chlamydial heat shock protein. Proceedings of the Eighth International Symposium on Human Chlamydial Infections. Orfila J et al (eds) Società Editrice Esculapio, Bologna, Italy, pp 502-505

27. Toye B, Laferriere C, Claman P, Jessamine P, Peeling R (1993) Association between antibody response to the chlamydial heat schock proteins and tubal infertility. J Infect Dis 168:1236-1240

Chapter 3   Laboratory Diagnosis

Francesco Blasi and Roberto Cosentini

Introduction

Chlamydia pneumoniae is a recently identified micro-organism frequently involved in respiratory tract infections and to a less degree in extrapulmonary diseases [1, 2].

The classification of *Chlamydia pneumoniae* among "new" and "emerging" pathogens is probably due to the rather difficult laboratory diagnosis which hampered the correct evaluation of its epidemiologic role. Laboratory diagnosis is based on culture, identification in biological specimens by means of monoclonal antibodies, polymerase chain reaction (PCR) and on serological methods.

In this chapter we describe and discuss the methods for culture isolation, direct antigen detection, PCR and specific antibody titre determination.

Isolation and culture

The first isolate of *Chlamydia pneumoniae* was obtained from the conjunctival swab of a Tawanese child, participating in a survey for thracoma vaccination in 1965 [3]. The culture was run in egg yolk sac. This culture method showed a low sensitivity for *C. pneumoniae* isolation and was therefore abandoned and other methods were developed. Several cell lines have been used; HeLa 229 and McCoy cells, used for other *chlamydiae*, showed a better sensitivity in comparison to egg yolk sac but proved suboptimal [4].

The human line HL cells, previously used for respiratory sincytial virus, present a high sensitivity for *C. pneumoniae* isolation and propagation [5].

In order to enhance the growth of *C. pneumoniae* various techniques are available. Kuo [6] indicates pretreatment of cell monolayers with DEAE-dextran (particularly for HeLa 229 cells), centrifugation of inoculum, and the addition of cycloheximide as host cell metabolic inhibitor. *C. pneumoniae* culture must be run at 35°C.

C. pneumoniae reticulate and elementary bodies can be detected by immunofluorescence using specific monoclonal antibodies (Fig. 1).

Specimens for *C. pneumoniae* culture can be obtained from many sources, including pharyngeal swab, sputum, bronchial aspirate or bronchoalveolar lavage, and pleural fluid. The handling and storage of specimens require particular care due to the thermolability of the organism. *C. pneumoniae* viability is affected by quick freezing even when stored in an optimal buffer such as SPG [6].

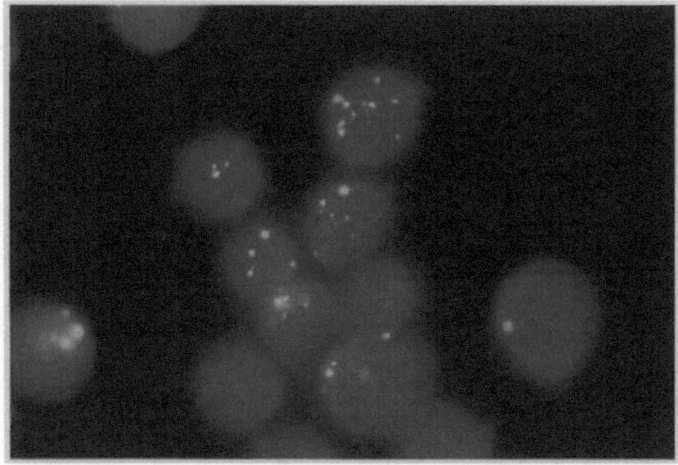

Fig. 1. *Chlamydia pneumoniae* reticulate and elementary bodies detected by immunofluorescence using specific monoclonal antibodies in a McCoy cell line

Other methods of detection

Indirect immunofluorescence tests for direct detection of *C. pneumoniae* organisms in clinical specimens have recently been developed. We have used two kits, one from Cellabs (Brookvale, Australia) and more recently one from DAKO (Ely, U.K.) using pharyngeal swab specimens (Fig. 2).

In our experience, the test sensitivity in presence of acute respiratory infections was around 20%, with a rather high specificity. False positive results may derive from non-specific background staining of mucus and other secretions.

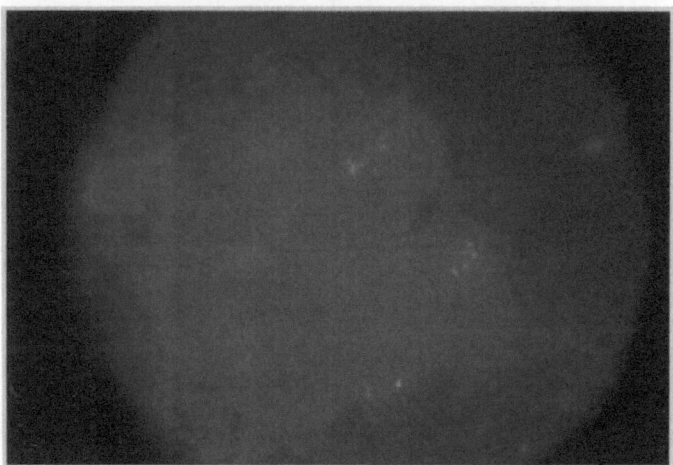

Fig. 2. Indirect immunofluorescence tests for direct detection of *Chlamydia pneumoniae* in pharyngeal swab specimen

Both these tests utilize a monoclonal antibody to *C. pneumoniae* that binds specifically to inclusions such as elementary bodies and reticulate bodies. A positive diagnosis is made when fixed stained pharyngeal specimens show at least four chlamydial elementary bodies. They appear as bright apple-green fluorescent pin-point, smooth edged disc shaped bodies with a diameter of approximately 300 nm. Reticulate bodies are 2-3 times larger than elementary bodies and they either fluoresce evenly or possess dark centers with a halo of fluorescence. A negative diagnosis is reported when fixed stained smears are free of chlamydial organisms but cells are present. We always run the test in duplicate.

Oheme [7] has recently reported the utility of gargle specimens for *C. pneumoniae* direct detection using this method. Recent reports indicate the possible role of polymerase chain reaction (PCR) in the diagnosis of *C. pneumoniae* infection [8, 9].

The relative complexity and high costs of this technique prevent its use on a large scale. However, PCR may be of great value in the study of the possible role of chronic *C. pneumoniae* infection in the etiopathogenesis of epidemiologically relevant diseases such as coronary artery disease [10].

Serology

The first serological test developed for diagnosis of chlamydial infection was complement fixation (CF) based on the lipopolysaccaride antigen. Presumptive diagnosis of *C. psittaci* infection was based on this test. However, CF is unable to distinguish between antibodies to *C. psittaci, trachomatis* and *pneumoniae*. Moreover, less than 30% of *C. pneumoniae* infections give rise to a positive CF test [11].

The microimmunofluorescence test described by Wang [12] has become the serological "gold standard" for *C. pneumoniae* infections. This test is highly specific and sensitive when compared with culture [1] and allows the determination of specific IgG, IgM and IgA serum fractions. The antibody pattern in response to infection is shown in Table 1.

Table 1. Serologic tests for detection of *Chlamydia pneumoniae* infection

MICRO-IF
Acute infection
Fourfold increase of IgG or IgA titre
IgM titre $\geq$ 1:16
IgG titre $\geq$ 1:512
IgA titre $\geq$ 1:256
Past infection
IgG titre $\geq$ 1:16 $\leq$ 1:512
IgA titre $\geq$ 1:16 < 1:256
Complement fixation (non-specific for *C. pneumoniae* and positive in less than 1/3 of infected subjects)
Acute infection
Fourfold titre rise
Titre > 1:64

Figures 3 and 4 show antibody response respectively to primary and secondary *C. pneumoniae* infection. Routine absorption of IgG before IgM testing is recommended to prevent false positive IgM results due to rheumatoid factor, particularly in older patients where the prevalence of rheumatoid factor is greater than 10% between 51 and 70 years of age [13].

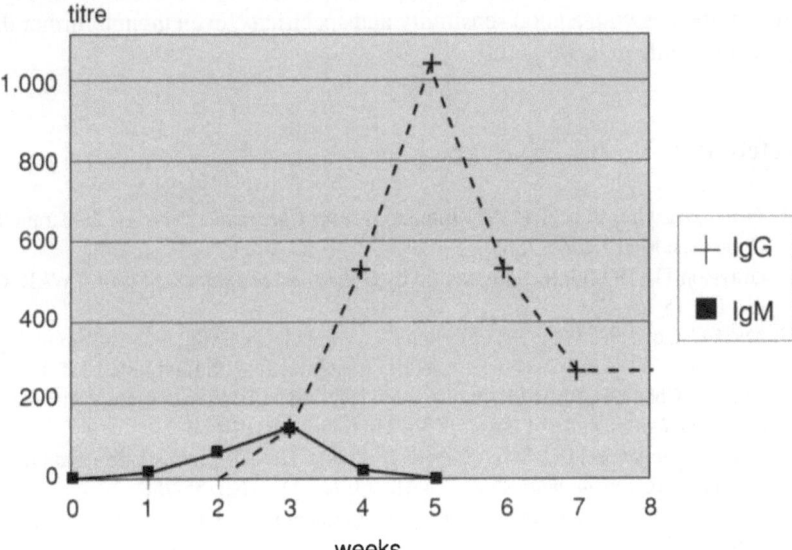

Fig. 3. Antibody response to *Chlamydia pneumoniae* primary infection

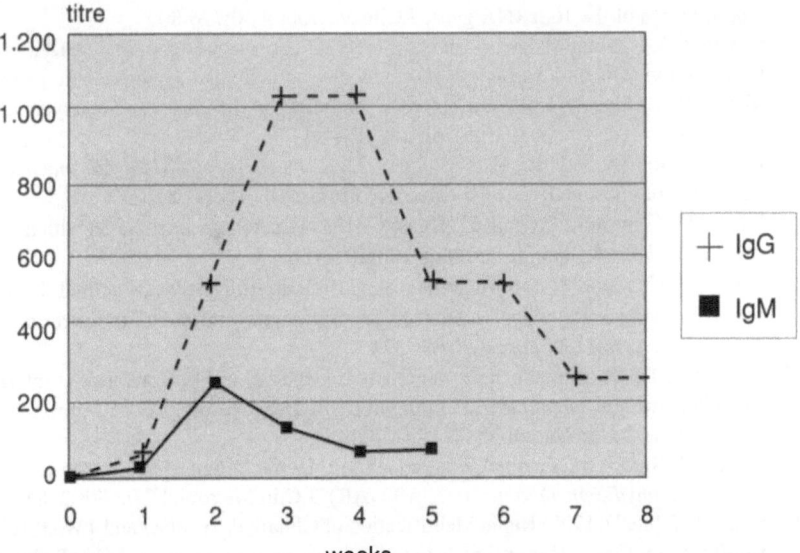

Fig. 4. Antibody response to *Chlamydia pneumoniae* secondary infection

C. pneumoniae specific antigen for micro-IF test can be purchased from The Washington Research Foundation, Seattle, USA. Commercial kits are available from Labsystems, Helsinki, Finland, and MRL Diagnostics, Cypress, USA. These kits are composed of slides dotted with three chlamydial antigens (*C. pneumoniae*, *C. trachomatis* and *C. psittaci*).

Other serological methods have recently been developed such as Enzyme immunoassay [14, 15]. This technique apparently allows the determination of IgG specific antibodies with a good sensitivity and specificity, even though further data are needed to confirm its reliability.

References

1. Thom DH, Grayston JT (1991) Infections with *Chlamydia pneumoniae* Strain TWAR. Clin Chest Med 12:245-256
2. Grayston JT (1992) Infections caused by *Chlamydia pneumoniae* Strain TWAR. Clin Infect Dis 15:757-763
3. Kuo CC, Chen HH, Wang SP, Grayston JT, Campbell LA (1986) A new *Chlamydia psittaci* strain called TWAR from acute respiratory tract infections. N Engl J Med 315:161-168
4. Kuo CC, Chen HH, Wang SP, Grayston JT (1986) Identification of a new group of *Chlamydia psittaci* strain called TWAR. J Clin Microbiol 24:1034-1037
5. Kuo CC, Grayston JT (1990) A sensitive cell line, HL cells, for isolation and propagation of *Chlamydia pneumoniae* strain TWAR. J Infect Dis 162:755-758
6. Kuo CC (1991) Culture and rapid methods in diagnosis of *Chlamydia pneumoniae* infections. In: Vaheri A, Tilton RC and Balows A (eds) Rapid methods and automation in microbiology and immmunology. Springer-Verlag, Berlin, pp 299-304
7. Oheme A, Rosler J (1992) Demonstration of *Chlamydia pneumoniae* in water used for gargling. Infection 20(1):56
8. Gaydos CA, Quinn TC, Eiden JJ (1992) Identification of *Chlamydia pneumoniae* by DNA amplification of the 16SrRNA gene. J Clin Microbiol 30:796-800
9. Gaydos CA, Roblin PM, Welsh LE et al (1992) Diagnostic utility of PCR-EIA and culture for detection of *Chlamydia pneumoniae* in symptomatic and asymptomatic patients. In: Mardh PA, La Placa M and Ward M (eds) Proceedings of the European Society for Chlamydia Research. The University of Uppsala p 244 A
10. Kuo CC, Shor A, Fukushi H et al (1993) Demonstration of *Chlamydia pneumoniae* in atherosclerotic lesion of coronary arteries. J Infect Dis 167(4):841-849
11. Marrie TJ, Grayston JT, Wang SP, Kuo CC (1987) Pneumonia associated with the TWAR strain of *Chlamydia*. Ann Intern Med 106:507-511
12. Wang SP, Grayston JT (1970) Immunologic relationship between genital TRIC, lymphogranuloma venereum, and related organisms in a new microtiter indirect immunofluorescence test. Am J Oftalmol 70:367-374
13. Verkooyen RP, Hazemberg MA, van Haaren GH et al (1992) Age-related interference with *Chlamydia pneumoniae* microimmunofluorescence serology due to circulating rheumatoid factor. J Clin Microbiol 30:1287-1290
14. Ladany S, Black CM, Farshy CE et al (1989) Enzyme immunoassay to determine exposure to *Chlamydia pneumoniae* (strain TWAR). J Clin Microbiol 27:2778-2783
15. Sillis M, White P (1990) Rapid identification of Chlamydia psittaci and TWAR (*C. pneumoniae*) in sputum samples using an amplified enzyme immunoassay. J Clin Pathol 43:260

Chapter 4   Epidemiology

ROBERTO COSENTINI, PAOLO TARSIA AND FRANCESCO BLASI

Introduction

Chlamydia pneumoniae has recently been recognized as a relevant cause of respiratory tract infections [1, 2]. It has been classified as a third species of *Chlamydia* genus by means of ultrastructural and DNA homology analysis [3].

C. *pneumoniae* is an obligate intracellular, gram-negative bacteria involved in a wide spectrum of respiratory tract infections; in fact, this agent can cause both upper respiratory tract infections - pharyngitis, sinusitis, and otitis - and lower respiratory tract infections, such as acute bronchitis, exacerbation of chronic bronchitis, and community-acquired and nosocomial pneumonias [4, 5, 6]. Several studies have recently stressed the importance of this agent in the development of respiratory diseases, showing a high incidence and prevalence of infections worldwide. Specific antibody prevalence in western countries is low in preschool children and climbs to over 50% in adults, remaining high in old age due to C. *pneumoniae* reinfection among adults [7].

In the present chapter we describe the general epidemiology of C. *pneumoniae* infection focusing on immunocompetent and immunocompromised populations in Italy.

Population Antibody Prevalence

Since the isolation of C. *pneumoniae* and the development of the specific microimmunofluorescence test, several seroepidemiological studies have been conducted both prospectively and retrospectively [8, 9]. These data have shown a worldwide diffusion of C. *pneumoniae* infection. In developed countries the infection seems to be rather uncommon before the age of 5; seroprevalence increases during school-age and reaches over 50% in adults. Males usually show a higher seropositivity rate. Our data [10] on Italian population are consistent with this trend.

Figure 1 shows seroprevalence in an immunocompetent population in Milan. A low prevalence (11%) in children under 10 years of age which progressively increases to 58% in adults over 70 years was observed. Males showed a higher prevalence at all ages with the exception of children under 10 years (-12%). The greatest difference (+21%) was observed in subjects between 50 and 59 years of age.

Seroepidemiological data from developing countries show an overall higher prev-

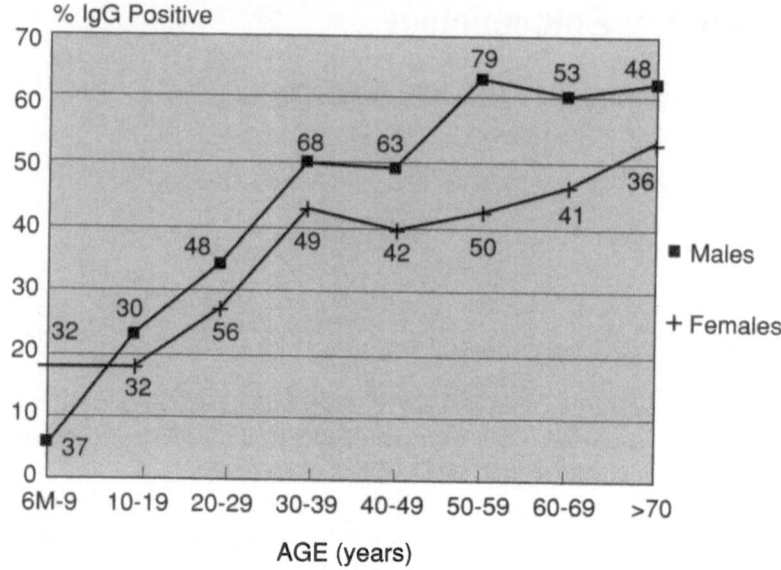

Fig. 1. *C. pneumoniae* seroprevalence in immunocompetent population in Milan, Italy. Numerical values indicate number of subjects

alence of *C. pneumoniae* infection [11]. In these populations preschool-age infection seems to be rather frequent and seroprevalence reaches more than 70% in adults.

In contrast to the numerous epidemiologic studies carried out in the general population, only limited data on *C. pneumoniae* infection in immunocompromised subjects are present in literature [12, 13, 14].

We have recently published preliminary results on *C. pneumoniae* seroprevalence in HIV-1 infected intravenous drug users and HIV-1 vertically infected children [10].

The seroprevalence of *C. pneumoniae* in the HIV-1 infected intravenous drug users (IDUs) was significantly higher ($p < 0.01$, chi-square test) than both HIV-1 negative IDUs and immunocompetent subjects matched for age and sex (Table 1). Four (4%) HIV-1 IDUs had an IgM titre >1:16, suggesting acute infection.

Children with vertically infected HIV-1 had a significantly higher prevalence ($p < 0.05$, Fisher's exact test) than healthy control subjects matched for age and sex (Table 2). Two (4%) HIV-1 children also showed IgM titre >1:16, suggesting acute infection.

Incidence of *Chlamydia pneumoniae* Infection

C. pneumoniae seems to be an important agent of respiratory tract diseases in humans. Several reports show a high incidence of infection in community-acquired pneumonia ranging from 6 to 25% and a remarkable role in pneumonia outbreaks in close communities like military garrisons, schools and families [8, 15-19]. Further-

Table 1. Demographic characteristics and serologic data in HIV-1 infected and HIV-1 negative injection drug users (IDUs) and in control subjects (C) matched for age and sex

	IDUs		C
	HIV-1 +ve (96)	*HIV-1 -ve* (126)	(147)
M/F	73/23	92/34	95/52
mean age (years)	29.1	29.6	28.5
age range (years)	18-35	18-37	18-34
IgG≥1:64	58 (60%)	41 (33%)	59 (40%)
IgM≥1:16	4 (4%)	0	0

+ve = positive; -ve = negative
$p < 0.01$ (chi-square test) *C. pneumoniae* seroprevalence in HIV-1 +ve Vs HIV-1-ve and Vs C
$p = 0.24$ (chi-square test) *C. pneumoniae* seroprevalence in HIV-1 -ve Vs C

Table 2. Demographic characteristics and serologic data of HIV-1 vertically infected children and control subjects matched for age and sex

	HIV-1 +ve (50)	Control (87)
M/F	23/27	42/45
age range (months)	8-123	6-120
IgG≥1:64	13 (26%)	9 (11%)
IgM≥1:16	2 (4%)	0

+ve = positive
$p < 0.05$ (Fisher's exact test) *C. pneumoniae* seroprevalence in HIV-1 +ve Vs Controls

more, *C. pneumoniae* is involved in upper respiratory tract infections (pharyngitis, sinusitis, otitis) and in acute exacerbations of chronic bronchitis [5, 6]. Recently, Hahn [20] has reported about a possible etiopathogenetic role of this pathogen in adult onset of asthma and in asthma exacerbation.

Since the identification of *C. pneumoniae*, several diseases associated with this infection, such as erythema nodosum, Guillain-Barré syndrome, culture negative endocarditis, thyroiditis, arthritis and encephalitis have been sporadically reported [21-23]. Seroepidemiologic evidence of a possible association between *C. pneumoniae* infection and sarcoidosis has also been reported [24].

Saikku [25, 26] and other Authors [27-29] have found an association between *C. pneumoniae* and coronary artery disease. This topic is extensively analysed elsewhere in this book (see Chap. 8).

Table 3 summarizes published data on the incidence of *C. pneumoniae* infections.

Periodicity

According to seroepidemiologic survey performed in western countries *C. pneumoniae* infection seems to be both endemic and epidemic [30]. Peaks of incidence (epidemic) generally last 2-3 years, although shorter outbreaks have been reported, whereas periods of low incidence last 3 - 4 years, suggesting an approximately 6-year cycle in the incidence of *C. pneumoniae* infection [1]. No evidence of seasonal periodicity has been observed [1].

Immunity

As outlined in Chap. 3 the serologic response to *C. pneumoniae* infection is characterised by two different patterns. Primary infection shows CF positivity and IgM titre rise followed by IgG increase, whereas reinfection shows IgG and IgA titre rise without IgM and CF increase.

Table 4 shows the timing of antibody response to *C. pneumoniae* infection. IgM antibodies are usually undetectable after 2-6 months from acute infection, whereas IgA may persist longer and could represent indirect evidence of persistent infection [31].

In immunocompetent subjects IgG antibodies may be detectable for more than two years [1], whereas in immunocompromised subjects with HIV-1 infection we have observed a shorter persistance (less than one year), probably due to the impaired antibody synthesis in the immunocompromised host [32].

Table 3. Incidence of *Chlamydia pneumoniae* infections

Disease	Range of incidence	References
Asymptomatic infection	Common	1
Flu-like syndrome	Common	1
Community-acquired pneumonia	6-25%	1, 2, 4, 9, 11, 35, 36
Outbreaks in close communities	–	8, 15, 32, 33
Family outbreaks	–	16, 17, 18, 19
High respiratory tract infections	5-10%	37, 38
COPD exacerbations	4- 5%	5, 6
Asthma attacks	1-18%	20

Table 4. Timing (weeks) of antibody response to *Chlamydia pneumoniae* infection

	IgM	IgG	IgA	CF
First infection	2-4	6-8	–	2-3
Reinfection	low titre if any	1-3	1-2	low titre if any

Transmission

Current available data suggest that *C. pneumoniae* is primarly trasmitted by human to human without any animal reservoir [8, 33]. Wang did not find any serological evidence of cat or dog infection during the Finnish military epidemics [34]. However, a recent paper indicate the remarkable degree of momp gene DNA homology (>97%) between the koala type-I strain of *C. psittaci* and *C. pneumoniae* raising some questions on the host specificity, classification and evolutionary relationship of the different chlamydial species [39].

    C. pneumoniae infection spreads slowly with a case-to-case interval of about 30 days. Serological data show that the duration of epidemics varies from 5 to 8 months, suggesting a relatively long incubation period.

    Family transmission, from child to child, has been observed in Japan in 1990 [16]; Mordhorst [17] described an outbreak of *C. pneumoniae* infections in four farm families living close together in Denmark, with an unusually high incidence of symptomatic infections, particularly lower respiratory tract infections, among family members. These data support the human-to-human contact spread of *C. pneumoniae* infection, and underline the role of this agent in family cluster respiratory infections, although Aldous [18], in a serologic study of family serum samples carried out betwen 1966 and 1979, reported that acute infections more often affected a single family member than multiple members.

    We recently reported two family outbreaks where we recorded a high rate (75%) of symptomatic infections [19]. These data are in contrast with the low incidence of infection recorded during epidemics in military trainees in Finland [8] and in the serologic study of Aldous [18], while they are consistent with those reported by Mordhorst [17]; the latter, in fact, observed a family cluster with relatively high rate of infection.

    The time span of infection spread in both families was unusually short, ranging from 5 to 18 days; this may be explained by their living habits. In fact, both families lived in small flats, with high person-to-person contact.

References

1. Thom DH, Grayston JT (1991) Infections with *Chlamydia pneumoniae* strain TWAR. Clin Chest Med 12:245-256
2. Marrie TJ (1993) *Chlamydia pneumoniae*. Thorax 48:1-4
3. Grayston JT, Kuo CC, Campbell LA, Wang SP (1989) *Chlamydia pneumoniae* sp. nov. for *Chlamydia* sp. strain TWAR. Int J Sys Bacteriol 39:88-90
4. Grayston JT, Campbell LA, Kuo CC, Mordhorst CH, Saikku P, Thom DH, Wang SP (1990) A new respiratory tract pathogen: *Chlamydia pneumoniae* strain TWAR. J Infect Dis 161:618-625
5. Beaty CD, Grayston JT, Wang SP, Kuo CC, Reto CS, Martin TR (1991) *Chlamydia pneumoniae* strain TWAR infection in patients with chronic obstructive pulmonary disease. Am Rev Respir Dis 144:1408-1410
6. Blasi F, Legnani D, Lombardo VM et al (1993) *Chlamydia pneumoniae* infection in acute-

exacerbations of COPD. Eur Respir J 6:19-22

7. Saikku P (1992) The epidemiology and significance of *Chlamydia pneumoniae*. J Infect 25:27-34

8. Kleemola M, Saikku P, Visakorpi R, Wang SP, Grayston JT (1988) Epidemics of pneumonia caused by TWAR, a new Chlamydia organism, in military trainees in Finland. J Infect Dis 157:230-236

9. Marrie TJ, Grayston JT, Wang SP, Kuo CC (1987) Pneumonia associated with TWAR strain of chlamydia. Ann Intern Med 106:507-511

10. Blasi F, Cosentini R, Clerici Shoeller M, Lupo A, Allegra L (1993) *Chlamydia pneumoniae* seroprevalence in immunocompetent and immunocompromised populations in Milan. Thorax 48:1261-1263

11. Saikku P, Ruutu P, Leinonen M, Panelius J, Tupasi TE, Grayston JT (1988) Acute lower-respiratory-tract infection associated with *Chlamydia* TWAR antibody in Filipino children. J Infect Dis 158:1095-1907

12. Augenbraun MH, Roblin MR, Chirwing K, Landman D, Hammerschlag MR (1991) Isolation of *Chlamydia pneumoniae* from lungs of patients infected with the human immonodeficiency virus. J Clin Microbiol 29:401-402

13. Clark R, Mushatt D, Fazal B (1991) Case Report: *Chlamydia pneumoniae* pneumonia in an HIV- infected man. Am J Med Sci 302(3):155-156

14. Gaydos CA, Flower CL, Gill VJ, Eiden JJ, Quinn TC (1993) Detection of *Chlamydia pneumoniae* by polymerase chain reaction-enzyme immunoessay in an immunocompromised population. Clin Infect Dis 17:718-723

15. Pether JVS, Wang SP, Grayston JT (1989) *Chlamydia pneumoniae* strain TWAR as the cause of an outbreak in a boys' school previously called *psittacosis*. Epidemiol Infect 103:395-400

16. Yamazaki T, Nakada H, Sakurai N, Kuo CC, Wang SP, Grayston JT (1990) Transmission of *Chlamydia pneumoniae* in young children in a Japanese family. J Infect Dis 162:1390-1392

17. Mordhorst CH, Wang SP, Grayston JT (1992) Outbreak of *Chlamydia pneumoniae* infection in four farm families. Eur J Clin Microbiol Infect Dis 11:617-620

18. Aldous MB, Grayston JT, Wang SP (1992) Seroepidemiology of *Chlamydia pneumoniae* TWAR infection in Seattle families, 1966-1979. J Infect Dis 166:646-649

19. Blasi F, Cosentini R, Denti F, Allegra L (1994) Two family outbreaks of *Chlamydia pneumoniae* infection. Eur Respir J 7:102-104

20. Hahn DL, Dodge RW, Golubjatnikov R (1991) Association of *Chlamydia pneumoniae* (strain TWAR) infection with wheezing, asthmatic bronchitis, and adult-onset asthma. JAMA 266:225-230

21. Bruu AL, Haukenes G, AAsen S, Grayston JT, Wang SP, Klausen OG, Myrmel H, Hasseltvedt V (1991) *Chlamydia pneumoniae* infections in Norway 1981-87 earlier diagnosed as ornithosis. Scand J Infect Dis 23:299-304

22. Haidl S, Ivarsson S, Bjerre I, Persson K (1992) Guillain-Barré syndrome after *Chlamydia pneumoniae* infection. N Engl J Med 326:576-577

23. Marrie TJ, Harczy M, Mann OE (1990) Culture-negative endocarditis probably due to *Chlamydia pneumoniae*. J Infect Dis 161:127-129

24. Groenhagen-Riska C, Saikku P, Riska H (1988) Antibodies to TWAR- a novel type of *Chlamydia* in sarcoidosis. In: Grassi C, Rizzato G, Pozzi E (eds) Sarcoidosis and granulomatous disorders. Elsevier Science Publishers, Amsterdam, pp 297-301

25. Saikku P, Leinonen M, Mattila K, Ekman MR, Nieminen MS, Makela PH, Huttunen JK, Valtonen V (1988) Serological evidence of an association of a novel *Chlamydia*, TWAR,

with coronary heart disease and acute myocardial infarction. Lancet ii:983-986

26. Saikku P, Leinonen M, Tenkanen L, Linnanmaki E, Ekman MR, Manninen V, Manttari M, Frick MH, Huttunen JK (1992) Chronic *Chlamydia pneumoniae* infection as a risk factor for coronary heart disease in the Helsinki Heart Study. Ann Intern Med 116:273-278

27. Shor A, Kuo CC, Patton DL (1992) Detection of *Chlamydia pneumoniae* in coronary arterial fatty-streaks and atheromatous plaques. S Afr Med J 82:158-161

28. Thom DH, Grayston JT, Siskovick DS, Wang SP, Weiss NS, Daling JR (1992) Association of prior infection with *Chlamydia pneumoniae* and angiographically demonstrated coronary artery disease. JAMA 268:68-72

29. Linnanmaki E, Leinonen M, Mattila K, Nieminen MS, Valtonen V, Saikku P (1993) Specific circulating immune complexes in patients with chronic coronary heart diseases. Circulation 87:1130-1134

30. Grayston JT (1992) Infections caused by *Chlamydia pneumoniae* strain TWAR. Clin Infect Dis 15:757-763

31. Saikku P (1991) Problems in diagnosis of chronic *Chlamydia pneumoniae* infections. In Vaheri A, Tilton RC, Balows A (eds) Rapid methods and automation in miscrobiology and immunology. Springer-Verlag , Berlin, pp 309-313

32. Blasi F, Boschini A, Cosentini R, Legnani D, Smacchia C, Ghira C, Allegra L (in press) Outbreak of *Chlamydia pneumoniae* infection in an ex injection-drug users community. Chest

33. Saikku P, Wang SP, Kleemola M, Brander E, Rusanen E, Grayston JT (1985) An epidemic of mild pneumonia due to an unusual *Chlamydia psittaci* strain. J Infect Dis 151:832-839

34. Wang SP, Grayston JT (1986) Microimmunofluorescence serological studies with TWAR organism. In: Oriel JD, Ridgway G, Schachter J, Taylor-Robinson D, Ward M (eds) Chlamydial infections. Cambridge University Press, Cambridge, pp 329-332

35. Fang GD, Fine M, Orloff J, Arisumi D et al (1990) New and emerging etiologies for community-acquired pneumonia with implications for therapy. Medicine 69:307-316

36. Blasi F, Cosentini R, Legnani D, Denti F, Allegra L (1993) Incidence of community-acquired pneumonia caused by *Chlamydia pneumoniae* in Italian patients. Eur J Clin Microbiol Infect Dis 12:696-699

37. Huovinen P, Lahtonen R, Ziegler T, Meurman O et al (1989) Pharyngitis in adults: the presence and the coexistence of viruses and bacterial organisms. Ann Intern Med 110:612-616

38. Ogawa H, Fujisawa T, Kazuyama Y (1990) Isolation of *Chlamydia pneumoniae* from middle ear aspirates of otitis media with effusion: a case report. J Infect Dis 162:1000-1001

39. Girjes AA, Carrick FN, Lavin MF (1994) Remarkable sequence relatedness in the DNA encoding the major outer membrane protein of *Chlamydia psittaci* (koala type-I) and *Chlamydia pneumoniae*. Gene 138 (1-2):139-142

Chapter 5 Pharmacological and Pharmacokinetic Basis of *Chlamydia pneumoniae* Treatment

GIULIANA GIALDRONI GRASSI

Introduction

Chlamydia pneumoniae, such as other *Chlamydia* species, is an obligate intracellular parasite. To inhibit its growth it is necessary that the antimicrobial agent penetrates cells and can interfere with protein synthesis of the micro-organism. Therefore antibiotics that are likely to be active against *Chlamydia pneumoniae* are macrolides, tetracyclines, chloramphenicol, quinolones and rifampicin, which have demonstrated the capacity to enter cells and develop antimicrobial activity intracellularly for *Chlamydia psittaci* and *Chlamydia trachomatis*, as well as for other pathogens.

Drugs

In order to exert their antibacterial activity, antibiotics must reach the infectious focus. Infection can be localized in the interstitial spaces of tissues or inside the cells. Drug physicochemical properties are the main factors conditioning their distribution in tissues and penetration in cells.

The capacity to enter cells is a prerequesite for activity of antibiotics in intracellular infections, particularly if the pathogen is an obligate intracellular parasite.

Clindamycin, rifampicin, macrolides and fluoroquinolones accumulate in phagocytes [1, 2]. Clindamycin reaches a cellular/extracellular (C/E) ratio of about 10, while rifampicin penetration is lower, with a C/E ratio of 2-3. Also tetracyclines and chloramphenicol penetrate to a moderate extent (C/E ratio 0.5-2). Fluoroquinolones accumulate in cytosol of phagocytes at C/E ratio of 2-8: both uptake and release are rapid. Macrolides show a great capacity of accumulation in phagocytes. They are localized in cytosol and lysosomes. In polymorphonuclear neutrophils C/E ratio varies from 2 to 14 for erythromycin and josamycin and reach the highest values for dirithromycin and azithromycin (Table 1) [3-8]. The C/E ratio of the former is about 80 and that of the latter can reach values over 200 [9, 10]. A peculiar behaviour is shown by azithromycin: it has a very long half-life of about 50 h accompained by very low serum levels and extremely high tissue and intracellular levels, particularly in PMN, alveolar macrophages and fibroblasts, from which it is slowly released [11].

Correlation between intracellular accumulation and antimicrobial activity has been submitted to careful analysis. Not always a large amount of antibiotics in cell

Table 1. Intracellular/extracellular concentration ratio of some macrolide derivatives in human PMN, AM and Fibroblast

Derivative	PMN	AM	Fibroblast
Erythromycin	2-14	15-40	35
Roxithromycin	14-22	60	
Clarithromycin	12	33	
Dirithromycin	83	nd	
Azithromycin	40-200	20->500	>1000

PMN = polymorphonuclear neutrophils; AM = alveolar macrophage; nd = not determined
References : 3, 4, 6, 9, 10, 18, 19

assures higher antibacterial activity. Cell penetration of macrolides correlates extracellular concentration and antimicrobial activity correlates intracellular accumulation in experimental models. Fluoroquinolones, which accumulate into cells to a lesser extent than macrolides, show nevertheless an excellent antimicrobial activity, while clindamycin, that shows a C/E ratio somewhat superior to fluoroquinolones, displays a scarce activity against intracellular *Staph. aureus* [3]. Evidently the nature of parasite, its growth rate, the different experimental conditions as well as the mechanism of action of the antibiotic can greatly influence the outcome of experiences performed *in vitro* and in animal models. The clinical efficacy showed in intracellular infections by antibiotics with the capacity to enter cell has confirmed, at least in the majority of cases, the good predictive property of some experimental models.

For the therapy of infections of respiratory tree, according to their localization, it is necessary that antibiotics reach adequate concentration in lung parenchima, bronchial tissue, bronchial secretions and inside the cells if infection is intracellular. In a schematic way it can be said that in lung and bronchial mucosa beta-lactams and aminoglycosides reach concentrations that are similar or somehow lower than in blood, while macrolides and quinolones attain levels higher than in blood. However, some marginal differences exist from derivative to derivative [12-15]. On the contrary profound differences exist among the different classes of antibiotics, and sometimes among derivatives belonging to the same antibiotic class, with regard to concentration in bronchial secretions and sputum. In fact, the penetration in these secretions implies the passage through a series of cellular membranes, proteinaceous material of different origin, bacterial debris, mucus etc, that has been defined as *haematobronchial barrier*. Determinants of the entity of passage are mainly the physicochemical properties of the drug, its degree of ionization as well as the degree of inflammation and tissue injury [16]. Usually beta-lactams penetrate very poorly in bronchial secretions, where they reach concentrations equal to 10-20% or less of serum levels [12, 13, 16]. Aminoglycosides concentrations represent 30-40% of serum levels. Quinolones and macrolides penetrate better, the former reaching levels equal to those of serum, the latter with levels that are 5-6 fold or even higher than those of serum [13, 17-19]. The recently developed *microlavage technique* performed by fibreoptic bronchoscopy allows to obtain specimen of alveolar epithelial lining fluid and alveolar macrophages in which it is possible to measure antibiotic concentrations [20].

The possibility to have these informations about the pharmacokinetic behaviour of antibiotics at level of the respiratory tract has been of great importance in anticipating and in assessing their clinical efficacy in respiratory infection. In particular, when dealing with infection due to obligate intracellular parasites, it can be expected that among antibiotics, whose intracellular penetration has been ascertained, there will be the derivative or the derivatives of choice for treatment of chlamydial infections.

In vitro Activity

Due to the obligate intracellular localization of *Chlamydia pneumoniae* the *in vitro* antibiotic susceptibility testing must be performed in tissue cultures. The determinations have been most commonly carried out on cultures of HEp-2 and HeLa 229 cells, but also McCoy and HL cells have been employed. The test is usually performed in 96 well microtiter plates, the inoculum being 0.1 ml of the test strain diluted to obtain 10^3 - 10^4 inclusion-forming units per ml. After incubation at 35°C for 72 h, cultures are fixed and stained for inclusions with fluorescein-conjugated antibody to the lipopolysaccharide genus antigen. The Minimal Inhibitory Concentration (MIC) is the lowest antibiotic concentration at which no inclusion is seen. The Minimal Chlamydiacidal Concentration (MCC) can be determined by aspirating the antibiotic containing medium from cell culture, carefully washing wells and adding antibiotic free medium. Cultures are then frozen at -70°C, thawed and passed onto new cells, incubated at 35°C for 72 h and then fixed and stained to detect inclusions. The MCC is the lowest antibiotic concentration at which no inclusion is detectable after passage [21, 22].

Data on *in vitro* activity of antibiotics against *C. pneumoniae* are limited, due to the difficulty in isolating the agent and performing the susceptibility test. Moreover, data in literature are often discrepant: probably results are influenced by the condition of experience. The timing of addition of the antibiotic to the culture is crucial: if it is added before inoculating *C. pneumoniae* in culture cells, MIC and MCC can be up to 8-fold lower than if it is added after *C. pneumoniae* inoculation. It has been pointed out that the tests in which cells are infected before being exposed to antibiotics are likely to be closer to conditions- existing *in vivo*, where infection preceeds always the administration of antibiotics (Table 2). However, not all antibiotics are affected to the same extent by this different conduct of experience [23].

Other factors that can lead to find somehow different MICs are the technique by which the test is carried out, namely in microtiter plates or tubes, and the difficulty in determining the exact breakpoint [24]. However, even if we compare studies carried out apparently in very similar conditions, we observe some evident discrepancies, the reason of which has not been clarified. Tetracyclines and erythromycin show a good *in vitro* activity and have been so far the drugs most commonly employed in the treatment of *C. pneumoniae* infection [25-29] (Table 3).

Table 2. MIC and MCC of some macrolides, tetracyclines and quinolones against *Chlamydia pneumoniae* in function of timing of antibiotic addition to cell culture

		Antibiotic added before cell infection		Antibiotic added after cell infection	
		MIC °	*MCC* *	*MIC* °	*MCC* *
		µg/ml		µg/ml	
Tetracycline	a)	0.5	0.5	0.5	>2
	b)	1			
Erythromycin	a)	0.12	1	0.5	>1
	b)	0.06			
Clarithromycin	a)	0.015	0.015	0.03	0.03
	b)	0.007			
Azithromycin	a)	1	2	0.5	2
	b)	0.5			
Ciprofloxacin	a)	2	2	16	16
	b)	2			
Sparfloxacin	a)	0.25	1	0.5	>2

a) data from Cooper et al [23]; b) data from Fenelon et al [28]; °MIC = Minimal Inhibitory Concentration; *MCC = Minimal Chlamydiacidal Concentration

The most active macrolides seem to be clarithromycin [23, 28-33]. This finding has been recently confirmed by the determination of susceptibility to clarithromycin in the largest series of recent clinical isolates of *C. pneumoniae* so far tested, during the course of a multicenter study carried out in USA, comparing clarithromycin and erythromycin in the treatment of community-acquired pneumonia in children (3-12 years of age). *C. pneumoniae* was isolated in 42 (16%) of the 260 children envolved. MIC_{90} and MCC_{90} of the 49 isolates that were tested, resulted to be 0.031 µg/ml and 0.031 µg/ml for clarithromycin, 0.125 µg/ml and 0.125 µg/ml for erythromycin respectively [34]. Also the 14-hydroxy-metabolite of clarithromycin mantains a good activity comparable to roxithromycin, azithromycin and erythromycin. Very few data exist on doxycycline, but it seems to be as active as tetracycline [23].

Fluoroquinolones show good activity: the most active compounds are sparfloxacin and BAY3118 followed by tosufloxacin and L-ofloxacin (Levofloxacin). L-ofloxacin is more active than ofloxacin [23, 29, 31, 32, 35-39]. Susceptibility of *Chlamydia pneumoniae* to ciprofloxacin and fleroxacin is lower than to other tested derivatives, but MIC≥16 µg/ml reported for ciprofloxacin by some Authors [23] seems to be excessively high (Table 4).

Beta-lactams and aminoglycosides which do not enter cells or enter very poorly and whose mechanism of action is directed to bacterial cell wall, a structure lacking in *Chlamydiae*, are inactive against them. However, Kuo and Grayston [25] observed that penicillin and ampicillin, while showing no activity on *Chlamydia* viability, could be effective in inhibiting infectivity. Rifampicin, clindamycin, chlorampheni-

Table 3. *In vitro* susceptibility of *C. pneumoniae* to Tetracyclines and Macrolides

Author [Ref. No.]	Tetracycline MIC° µg/ml	Tetracycline MCC* µg/ml	Doxycycline MIC° µg/ml	Doxycycline MCC* µg/ml	Erythromycin MIC° µg/ml	Erythromycin MCC* µg/ml	Clarithromycin MIC° µg/ml	Clarithromycin MCC* µg/ml	14OH-Clarithromycin MIC° µg/ml	14OH-Clarithromycin MCC* µg/ml	Azithromycin MIC° µg/ml	Azithromycin MCC* µg/ml	Roxithromycin MIC° µg/ml	Roxithromycin MCC* µg/ml
Kuo (1988) [25]	0.05-0.1	0.05-0.1			0.01-0.05	0.01-0.05								
Chirgwin (1989) [29]	0.125	0.06-0.125			0.06-0.125	0.125	0.015-0.03	0.03			0.06-0.125	0.125-0.25	0.125	0.125
Fenelon (1990) [28]	1		0.25		0.06		0.007				1		0.25	
Ridgway (1991) [33]					0.06		0.007				0.5		0.25	
Cooper (1991) [23]	0.5	>2			0.5	>1	0.03	0.03	0.03	0.25	0.5	2		
Welsh (1992) [22] a)	0.125-1	0.125-2			0.125-0.25	0.25-1					0.125-0.25	0.25-1		
Welsh (1992) [22] b)	0.25-0.5	1-4			0.06-0.125	0.25-1					0.125-0.25	0.25		
Hammerschlag (1992) [31]			0.06-0.25	0.125-0.25	0.06-0.25	0.06-0.25	0.004-0.03	0.008-0.03			0.06-0.25	0.06-0.25		
Orfila (1992) [30]			0.01	1			0.25				2		0.05	
Roblin (1994) [34]					0.016-0.125	0.016-0.25	0.004-0.25	0.004-0.25						
Soejima (1994) [32]			0.015 °°				0.015							

°MIC = Minimal Inhibitory Concentration; *MCC = Minimal Chlamydiacidal Concentration (see text) (values are given as range of MIC or MCC against different strains or as value against type strain of *C. pneumoniae*); a) test in HeLa cells; b) test in HL cells; °° value for minocycline

Table 4. *In vitro* susceptibility of *C. pneumoniae* to Quinolones

Author [Ref. No.]	Ciprofloxacin MIC° μg/ml	Ciprofloxacin MCC* μg/ml	Ofloxacin MIC° μg/ml	Ofloxacin MCC* μg/ml	L-Ofloxacin MIC° μg/ml	L-Ofloxacin MCC* μg/ml	Lomefloxacin MIC° μg/ml	Lomefloxacin MCC* μg/ml	Sparfloxacin MIC° μg/ml	Sparfloxacin MCC* μg/ml	Fleroxacin MIC° μg/ml	Fleroxacin MCC* μg/ml	New Quinolones MIC° μg/ml	New Quinolones MCC* μg/ml
Chirgwin (1989) [29]	1	1												
Fenelon (1990) [28]	2		1				4				2			
Cooper (1991) [23]	16	>16												
Orfila (1990, 1992) [35, 37]			0.25				0.25		<0.01					
Hammerschlag (1992) [36]	0.25	0.25	0.5	0.5					0.06	0.06	2	2		
Hammerschlag (1992) [31]	-4	-8	-2	-2	0.125 / -0.5	0.125 / -0.5			0.125 / -0.25	0.125 / -0.5	-8	-8		
Andrews (1993) [38]	1	1											BAY3118 0.015	0.015
Roblin (1994) [39]			0.5	0.5					0.06	0.06			OPC-17116 0.25-0.5	0.5-2
Soejima (1994) [32]	1		0.5						0.063				Tosufloxacin 0.125	

°MIC = Minimal Inhibitory Concentration; *MCC = Minimal Chlamydiacidal Concentration (see text)

col and co-trimoxazole which show some *in vitro* activity against *C. trachomatis* and *C. psittaci*, could be active also against *C. pneumoniae*, but no data are so far available.

Clinical Relevance of Experimental Findings

The clinical efficacy of the different antibiotics in the treatment of *C. pneumoniae* infection is extensively treated in Chap. 6. It is worthwhile to observe that a good correlation between experimental data and clinical results seems to exist. Tetracyclines have been so far the most frequently prescribed drugs, leading to satisfactory clinical results [26, 27]. Some Authors complain that, in some cases, persistent positive cultures were obtained despite long courses (up to 30 days) of tetracyclines.

Some of the most recent fluoroquinolones and macrolide derivatives showed an excellent activity *in vitro* but, at present, it is not possible to give any clinical comparative evaluation. There are limited clinical experiences with ofloxacin: results were satisfactory [41, 42]. Sparfloxacin, one of the most active fluoroquinolones, showed an excellent activity in the experimental pneumonia caused by *C. pneumoniae* in leukopenic mice [43]. Clinical data are still scanty, but satisfactory [32, 44].

The macrolide derivative clarithromycin is one of the most active compound *in vitro*. However, some preliminary results seem to indicate that its clinical activity is equivalent to that of erythromycin. It is not possible to draw any definite conclusion from these findings. However, it seems of importance the observation that the persistence of *C. pneumoniae* in patients treated with either antibiotics did not appear to be secondary to the development of antibiotic resistance [34].

References

1. Johnson JD, Hand WL, Francis JB, King-Thompson NK, Corwin RW (1980) Antibiotic uptake by alveolar macrophages. J Lab Clin Med 95:429-439
2. Prokesch RC, Hand WL (1982) Antibiotic entry into polymorphonuclear leukocytes. Antimicrob Agents Chemother 21:373-380
3. Tulkens PM (1991) Intracellular pharmacokinetics and localization of antibiotics as predictors of their efficacy against intraphagocytic infections. Scand J Infect Dis [Suppl 74]:209-217
4. Tulkens PM (1991) Intracellular distribution and activity of antibiotics. Eur J Clin Infect Dis 10(2):100-106
5. Peters DH, Clissod SP (1992) Clarithromycin. A review of its antimicrobial activity, pharmacokinetic property and therapeutic potential. Drugs 44:117-164
6. Carlier MB, Zenebergh A, Tulkens PM (1987) Cellular uptake and subcellular distribution of roxithromycin and erythromycin in phagocytic cells. J Antimicrob Chemother 20 [Suppl B]:47-56
7. Fraschini F, Scaglione F, Pintucci, G Maccarinelli G et al (1991) The diffusion of clarithromycin and roxithromycin into nasal mucosa, tonsil and in lung in humans. J Antimicrob Chemother 27 [Suppl A]:61-65

8. Bergogne-Bérézin E (1993) Tissue distribution of dirithromycin: comparison with erythromycin. J Antimicrob Chemother 31 [Suppl C]:77-87
9. Anderson R, Joone G, van Rensburg CEJ (1988) An *in vitro* evaluation of the cellular uptake and intraphagocytic bioactivity of clarithromycin (A-56268, TE-031), a new macrolide antimicrobial agent. J Antimicrobial Chemother 22:923-933
10. MacDonald PJ, Pruul H (1991) Phagocyte uptake and transport of azithromycin. Eur J Clin Microbiol Infect Dis 10:828-833
11. Foulds G, Shepard RM, Johnson RB (1990) The pharmacokinetics of azithromycin in human serum and tissues. J Antimicrob Chemother 25 [Suppl A]:73-82
12. Bergogne-Bérézin E (1981) Penetration of antibiotics into the respiratory tree. J Antimicrob Chemother 8:171-174
13. Smith BR, LeFrock JL (1983) Bronchial tree penetration of antibiotic. Chest 83(6):904-908
14. Valcke Y, Pauwels R, Van Den Straeten M (1990) Pharmacokinetics of antibiotics in the lung. Eur Respir J 3:715-722
15. Baldwin DR, Honeybourne D, Wise R (1992) Pulmonary disposition of antimicrobial agents: *in vivo* observations and clinical relevance. Antimicrob Agents and Chemother 36(6):1176-1180
16. Gialdroni Grassi G (1980) Passaggio degli antibiotici nelle secrezioni bronchiali. In: Gialdroni Grassi G and Grassi C (eds). Aggiornamenti di chemioterapia. La Goliardica Pavese Publ., Pavia, pp 68-88
17. Gerdin DN, H.H.J.A (1989) Tissue penetration of the new quinolones in humans. Rev Infect Dis 11 [Suppl 5]:S1046-S1057
18. Baldwin DR, Wise R , Andrews JM, Ashby JP et al (1990) Azithromycin concentrations at the sites of pulmonary infection. Eur Respir J 3:886-890
19. Andrews JM, Honeybourne D, Greaves I, Baldwin D et al (1992) Clarithromycin levels in human bronchial mucosa, alveolar macrophages and serum. 8th Mediterranean Congress of Chemotherapy Athens, Greece Abs. 714
20. Baldwin DR, Honeybourne D, Wise R (1992) Pulmonary disposition of antimicrobial agents: methodological consideration. Antimicrob Agents Chemother 36:1171-1175
21. Gump DW (1991) Antimicrobial susceptibility testing for some atypical microrganisms: *Chlamydiae*, Mycoplasms, Rickettsia, and Spirochetes. In: Lorian V (ed) Antibiotic in laboratory medicine. 3rd Ed, Williams & Wilkins, pp 279-294
22. Welsh LE, Gaydos CA, Quinn TC (1992) *In vitro* evaluation of activities of azithromycin, erythromycin and tetracyclines against *Chlamydia trachomatis* and *Chlamydia pneumoniae*. Antimicrob Agents Chemother 36:291-294
23. Cooper MA, Baldwin D, Matthews RS, Andrews JM, Wise R (1991) *In vitro* susceptibility of *Chlamydia pneumoniae* (TWAR) to seven antibiotics. J Antimicrob Chemother 2:407-413
24. Roblin PM, Hammerschlag MR (1990) *In vitro* activity of sparfloxacin (CI-978, AT 4140) and other quinolones against *Chlamydia trachomatis* and *Chlamydia pneumoniae*. 30th Interscience Conference on Antimicrobial Agents and Chemotherapy, ICAAC, Atlanta Abs 22
25. Kuo CC, Grayston JT (1988) *In vitro* drug susceptibility of *Chlamydia* sp. strain TWAR. Antimicrob Agents Chemother 32:257-258
26. Atmar RL, Greenberg SB (1989) Pneumonia caused by *Mycoplasma pneumoniae* and the TWAR agent. Seminars in Respiratory Infections 4:19-31
27. Bourke SJ (1993) Chlamydial respiratory infections. British Med J 306:1219-1220
28. Fenelon LE, Mumtaz G, Ridgway GL (1990) The *in vitro* susceptibility of *Chlamydia pneumoniae*. J Antimicrob Chemother 26:763-767

29. Chirwing K, Roblin PM, Hammerschlag MR (1989) *In vitro* susceptibilities of *Chlamydia pneumoniae* Antimicrob Agents Chemother 1634-1635

30. Orfila J, Haider F (1992) *In vitro* susceptibilities of *Chlamydia pneumoniae* strain IOL 207 against clarithromycin, compared to different molecules. In: Adam D, Lode H, Rubinstein E (eds) Recent Advances in Chemotherapy. Proceedings of the 17th International Congress of Chemotherapy Berlin, Futuramed Publisher, Munich, Germany, pp 2454-2455

31. Hammerschlag MR, Qumei KK, Roblin PM (1992) *In vitro* activities of azithromycin, clarithromycin, L-ofloxacin and other antibiotics against *Chlamydia pneumoniae*. Antimicrob Agents Chemother 36:1573-1574

32. Soejima R, Niki Y, Kishimoto T, Kimura M, Kubota Y (1994) Anti-chlamydial activities of newly developed fluoroquinolones and their clinical usefulness for *Chlamydia* respiratory infections. 5th Int Symposium on new quinolones, Singapore, Abs 135

33. Ridgway GL, Mumtaz G, Fenelon L (1991) *In vitro* activity of clarithromycin and other macrolides against the type strain of *Chlamydia pneumoniae*. J Antimicrob Chemother 27 [Suppl A]:43-45

34. Roblin PM, Montalban G, Hammerschlag MR (1994) Susceptibilities of isolates of *Chlamydia pneumoniae* from children with pneumonia to clarithromycin and erythromycin. 2nd International Conference on the macrolides, azalides and streptogamins, Venice, Italy, Abs 150

35. Orfila F, Haider F (1990) *In vitro* susceptibility of *Chlamydia pneumoniae* (strain IOL 207) against a new fluoroquinolone, sparfloxacin, compared to different other molecules. 30th Interscience Conference on Antimicrobial Agents and Chemotherapy, ICAAC, Atlanta, Georgia, October 21-24, 1990, Abs 18

36. Hammerschlag MR, Hyman CL, Roblin PM (1992) *In vitro* activities of five quinolones against *Chlamydia pneumoniae*. Antimicrob Agents Chemother 36:682-683

37. Orfila J, Haider F (1992) *In vitro* susceptibility of *Chlamydia pneumoniae* strain IOL 207 against temafloxacin compared to different other molecules. In: Adam D, Lode H, Rubinstein E (eds) Recent Advances in Chemotherapy. Proceedings of the 17th International Congress of Chemotherapy, Berlin 1991, vol II, pp 2344-45, Futuramed Publisher, Munich, Germany

38. Andrews JM, Wise R, Brenwald N (1993) *In vitro* activity of BAY3118. VI Eur Congress Clin Microbiol and Infect Dis, Seville, March 28-31, 1993, Abs 4

39. Roblin PM, Montalban G, Hammerschlag MR (1994) *In vitro* activities of OPC-17116, a new quinolone, ofloxacin and sparfloxacin against *Chlamydia pneumoniae*. Antimicrob Agents Chemother 38:1402-1403

40. Dumornay W, Mandel L, Smith P, Schacter J (1992) Persistent infection with *Chlamydia pneumoniae* following acute respiratory illness. Clin Infect Dis 14:178-182

41. Kobayashi H (1986) Clinical evaluation of ofloxacin in lower respiratory tract infections. Infection 14 [Suppl 4]:S279-S282

42. Lipsky BA, Tack KJ, Kuo CC, Wang SP (1990) Ofloxacin treatment of *Chlamydia pneumoniae* (strain TWAR) lower respiratory tract infections. Am J Med 89:722-724

43. Nakata K, Okazaki Y, Hattori H, Nakamura S (1994) Protective effect of sparfloxacin in experimental pneumonia caused by *Chlamydia pneumoniae* in leukopenic mice. Antimicrob Agents Chemother 38:1757-1762

44. Aubier M, Garau J, Geslin P, Grassi C, Hosie G, Huchon G, Legakis N, Lode H, Regamey C and the European Study Group (1994) Sparfloxacin: an empiric therapy in community-acquired pneumonia. A meta-analysis of two comparative studies. 6th Int Congress for Infect Dis, Prague, April 26-30, 1994, Abs 459

Chapter 6   Clinical Characteristics of *Chlamydia pneumoniae* Infection

Francis P.V. Maesen and Benjamin I. Davies

Introduction

The symptoms of *Chlamydia pneumoniae* infection are mostly derived from case reports and descriptions of outbreaks in which the diagnosis of infection has been made
from the results of serological tests showing either high or rising titers of antibody to *C.
pneumoniae*, suggesting that the patients had suffered from an acute or an asymptomatic form of respiratory infection. The micro-immunofluorescence test showing IgM and
IgG antibodies is considered the golden standard in the serology of these infections. A
fourfold rise in IgM antibody titers or a single titer of 1:16 or greater are considered
evidence of recent infection as it is a single IgG titer > 1:512. If the IgM antibody titer
is negative and the IgG titer is between 1:16 and 1:512 it is generally supposed that the
patient has had an infection with *C. pneumoniae* in the past [3]. If the relatively insen-
sitive complement fixation test (CFT) technique has been used with the non-specific
genus antigen then an infection is assumed if there is a fourfold rise in serum antibody
titer in the course of a period of 10 days to 4 weeks, and certainly if the CFT titer is
greater than 1:64. Sometimes the patients fail completely to mount any form of complement fixing antibody response [8].

Respiratory Infections

Acute Infections

Acute infections with *C. pneumoniae* are the result either of a primary infection or a
reinfection. The latter is found mostly in adult patients despite the presence in the
serum of IgG antibodies, elicited by a previous infection which does not seem to
confer much immunity. Infections are transmitted by water droplet nuclei from the
respiratory tracts of infected persons: the human being is the only recognised source
of this micro-organism. This contrasts with *C. psittaci* for which all kinds of birds
can act as a reservoir.

   C. pneumoniae can also be differentiated from *C. trachomatis* by the fact that
infections with the former agent are not transmitted sexually and generally occur in
epidemics or endemic clusters.

   During epidemics, other infected patients are those who act as the source of
infection. The forming of clusters can clearly be seen when one sick patient is present

in closed communities such as barracks, student halls of residence or in large families [5, 6] and numerous secondary patients then become infected. Epidemics of *C. pneumoniae* infection have been described in many countries since 1986, the first being reported in Scandinavian recruits [16]. The infections were originally diagnosed as psittacosis even though there was no obvious avian source. Only later was it shown serologically that these infections were associated with a rise in antibody titers against *C. pneumoniae* [25]. Shortly afterwards, similar epidemics of infection were described in the USA, Philippines, Canada and various European countries (1,10, 23, 24, 27, 34). Epidemics seem to occur in cycles with a periodicity of 3 to 4 years [31]. They generally last 6 to 8 months and, unlike influenza epidemics, are not bound to any particular season.

Epidemics of *chlamydia* infection are likely to occur in low socio-economic groups, heavily populated districts, lifestyles such as those found in barracks and student halls, and in persons with reduced resistance, e.g. those who are malnourished or in the elderly. Frequent use of penicillin and cotrimoxazole for respiratory tract infections in developing countries seems to promote the spread of epidemics because neither agent is active against *C. pneumoniae* [27]. In comparison with viral respiratory tract infections the incubation time is rather long: 26 to 101 days [23]. According to some Authors, the average is 31 days as shown by epidemiological observations within families or communities [31].

Sero-epidemiological studies suggest that asymptomatic infections, that is to say positive *C. pneumoniae* cultures or positive direct immuno-fluorescence tests and positive serology without any clinical symptoms, are encountered more frequently than symptomatic infections and there is a greater chance of infection outside the home than within the family [5, 23]. Moreover, epidemiological studies have suggested that *C. pneumoniae* particularly affects the adolescent age-range [5, 29], so that most patients (40-50 %) suffer their primary infection between 5 and 15 years of age. Infections in elderly patients are generally reinfections. The incidence of infection in small children is relatively low and the disease is seldom encountered before the fifth year of life.

Developing countries such as Taiwan and the Philippine islands seem to be exceptional in this respect: up to 10 % of children under 5 years of age appear to have had *C. pneumoniae* infections in a poorly fed and densely populated district [5].

Symptoms of Acute Respiratory Infections

As a rule, acute infections progress in a biphasic manner when they are not treated or when treatment is inadequate. After an incubation period of approximately one month, symptoms develop in a way which suggests influenza: unproductive cough or the production of slightly yellowish mucoid sputum, sore throat, pain on swallowing and a hoarse voice. This last symptom is particularly indicative of chlamydial infections and may form an important aspect in differentiating them from influenza and from *Mycoplasma pneumoniae* infections. Body temperature is generally slightly increased reaching 38-39°C, seldom going higher. Muscle pain may develop particularly in the chest and intercostal muscles. The symptoms generally disappear slowly without therapy although an annoying but unproductive cough may sometimes last for months. Occasionally, after an initial period with an unproductive cough, the patient begins to produce mucopurulent or even frankly purulent sputum. If adequate treatment is given (for example with a tetracycline or erythromycin) the symptoms disappear very quickly even if they have been present for several months. After 10 days, and sometimes directly after the first phase of upper respiratory tract symptoms, the patient may develop shivering attacks followed by a new temperature peak of approximately 38.5 to 39°C and a pneumonic infiltrate is found. This may be accompanied by myalgic pain.

Pneumonia associated with *C. pneumoniae* accounts in all probability for up to 20% of all patients with acute community acquired pneumonia [22, 31]. The spectrum of the severity of the disease is enormous, varying from a short lived "common cold" to pneumonia severe enough to warrant admission to hospital.

Physical examination seldom shows abnormalities and there is generally no specific finding on percussion. In accordance with the small size of the individual pulmonary infiltrates as shown on the chest X-ray, localised fine rhonchi may be noted on auscultation. Sometimes there is cervical lymphadenopathy [10]. In both first and second phases the ESR is slightly raised (35 to 60 mm) and there is generally a slight leucocytosis with a shift to the left. Leucopenia has not been described. An accompanying maxillary sinusitis is very seldom found, usually at a much lower frequency than that observed with *M. pneumoniae* infections.

The chest X-ray shows multiple infiltrates but lobar pneumonia is very seldom encountered. The infiltrates are often segmental but are more usually sub-segmental [20]. Occasionally, segments of various different lobes can be involved and there is a general preference for both lower lobes. Atelectasis of lung segments and lobes can occasionally be found. Reactive pleurisy is rare and mostly not extensive.

The progress of the second phase of the acute infection is usually mild. Given that establishing the diagnosis of *C. pneumoniae* infection is not simple [8] and may be time consuming (up to two or three weeks), the diagnosis is mostly possible only on clinical grounds. This does not facilitate rapid or accurate diagnosis or the prescription of suitable treatment. It is thought [33] that the pneumonic infiltrates disappear rapidly and spontaneously even when no adequate therapy is given. This has been our experience in a clinical trial in which patients with radiologically confirmed community acquired pneumonia were treated with intramuscular injections of cefodizime or ceftriaxone, new third generation cephalosporins. In this series of 153 patients, raised ELISA titers against *C. pneumoniae* were recorded in 47 cases (31 %). These patients recovered within one or two weeks with practically no complications although the two antibiotics mentioned would not appear to be drugs of choice for the treatment of chlamydial infections [21].

C. pneumoniae generally causes a very mild disease in adults and younger patients. Several studies [29, 31] have shown a high prevalence of serum conversion in the age-range from 5 to 15 years, but it has not been possible to associate these serological findings directly with previous episodes of acute respiratory infection. In older patients, especially those who are poorly nourished or alcoholics, and in patients with chronic bronchitis, the picture can be confused by the development of superinfections mostly with either *Haemophilus influenzae* and/or *Streptococcus pneumoniae* [20]. Among our own hospitalized patients with acute community acquired pneumonia, 15 of the 47 with high ELISA antibody titers against *C. pneumoniae* also yielded positive sputum cultures (*S. pneumoniae* and *H. influenzae* 6 each, both these organisms in one patient, and *P. aeruginosa* in two others). Twelve of these 15 patients had pre-existing chronic bronchitis. Of the 32 yielding negative cultures, the sputum was grossly purulent in 18 of whom 11 had chronic bronchitis. Several instances of death as a result of complications of *C. pneumoniae* infections have been described [20].

There are indications that acute *C. pneumoniae* infections can play a role in the development of exacerbations of COPD [3, 7]. Several Authors [33, 34] have presented data in which 4-5 % of patients with acute exacerbations of COPD have shown serological evidence of acute *C. pneumoniae* infections and approximately 60 % of patients with exacerbations of chronic bronchitis have shown specific IgG titers as opposed to only 46 % in a matched group of controls [7]. This may suggest that infections with *C. pneumoniae* could also play a role in bringing about asthma and COPD during middle age [14]. A single case of severe pneumonia in a patient undergoing artificial ventilation has been associated with *C. pneumoniae*: infection by this agent was proven by culturing material obtained by bronchoalveolar lavage. Although the progress of the disease was complicated by respiratory insufficiency the patient responded well to tetracycline therapy [24]. The symptoms of acute pneumonia due to *C. pneumoniae* mostly disappear within 3 weeks but may recede earlier if treatment has been adequate. However, recurrences of a common cold-like illness with cough and recurrences of pneumonia have been described several weeks after apparent cure. Serological studies have suggested that these recurrences may be based on a new infection or on reactivation of an existing infection [16, 25].

Asymptomatic Carriers, Latent Infections

Carriers are asymptomatic patients in whom *C. pneumoniae* can be cultured from the throat or in whom the specific direct immunofluorescence test for this organism is positive in exudates from the nose or the throat. The serum contains specific antibody titers consistent with an acute infection but there are no clinical manifestations. It is probable that such patients with chronic carriage of *C. pneumoniae* are a very effective source of infection. Just as with *C. trachomatis*, patients have been found to yield positive cultures for *C. pneumoniae* despite treatment with macrolide antibiotics for many months [31]. Possible reactivation of latent infections has been described in patients admitted to a traumatology department where they underwent surgical operations [11].

Chronic cardiovascular disease and *Chlamydia pneumoniae*

There are indications that chronic infections with *C. pneumoniae* may be the basic aetiological factor in many patients with culture-negative endocarditis [19], chronic coronary arterial disease [12] and even in those with acute myocardial infarctions [18, 26]. There are also indications that unexpected and sudden death of young athletes may be connected with myocarditis associated with *C. pneumoniae* [35]. At autopsy small foci have been found in the heart muscle containing lymphocytic infiltrates and degenerative changes in the myocytes, as well as patchy fibrosis in the left ventricle and in the interventricular septum. In these patients, serological studies showed a recent *C. pneumoniae* infection, and test results for all other viral and chlamydial infections were negative.

The relation between chronic *C. pneumoniae* infection and coronary arterial disease has been suggested by the finding of a significantly higher frequency of *C. pneumoniae* infections in patients than in controls. This may be explained by the binding of chlamydial lipopolysaccharides to low density lipoproteins which may become immunogenic as a result of this modification and subsequently toxic for endothelial cells. Modified or antibody-associated low density lipoproteins cause the formation of foamy cells in vitro and this can be considered as the first phase in the development of the atherosclerotic process. *Chlamydiae* and their lipopoysaccharide components are equally potent inducers of tumor necrosis factor (TNF) which inhibits the lipoprotein lipase. This may lead to changes in lipid metabolism and accumulation of triglycerides in the blood [21, 28]. Recent studies have shown that there is a significant correlation between antibodies to *C. pneumoniae* and the extent of angiographically proven coronary arterial lesions [32]. Some Authors have suggested that the majority of patients with chronic coronary arterial disease are also suffering from chronic *C. pneumoniae* infection and that the chlamydia components have easy access to the circulation and thereafter can form complexes with previously existing antibodies [18]. More exact studies have been carried out by Shor et al [28] who found pear-shaped elementary bodies typical of the TWAR, or *C. pneumoniae* organism in atheromatous lesions using an ultramicroscopic technique.

Other Special Forms of *Chlamydia pneumoniae* Infection

Just as the case with viral and mycoplasma infections, some cases of erythema nodosum have been described in several patients in the course of *C. pneumoniae* infection [9]. Recent publications included a case of meningitis, hepatitis, iritis and erythema nodosum in one person with serologically proven acute *C. pneumoniae* infection [39] whereas another article has described a 13 years old previously healthy boy who developed the Guillain-Barré syndrome during serologically proven *C. pneumoniae* infection. In contrast, this infection does not seem to have any relation to the so called Chronic Fatigue Syndrome (CFS) [17].

Treatment of *Chlamydia pneumoniae* Infections

There is a generally expressed preference in literature for tetracycline or doxycycline. As a rule, a daily dosage of 2 g of tetracycline for 7-10 days is advised although others opt for 1g tetracycline for 21 days [2, 11]. Correct therapy with tetra-cycline may well depress the antibody response suggesting fairly rapid death of the causative micro-organism [16]. Erythromycin has also been prescribed at a dosage of 1 g daily for 10 days although various Authors are not in agreement over the results [2].

In vitro studies have shown that azithromycin and clarithromycin are also active against *C. pneumoniae*, as well as the more recent quinolone agents such as ofloxacin, L-ofloxacin and ciprofloxacin. This last drug has also been succesfully employed *in vivo* [7]. Clarithromycin seems to yield the lowest minimum inhibitory concentra-tions *in vitro* and may possibly be preferred to azithromycin which has an activity comparable to that of doxycycline, erythromycin, ofloxacin and L-ofloxacin [15]. There has been no concrete evidence yet that these newer (and more expensive) antimicrobial agents yield better results in the treatment of *C. pneumoniae* infec-tions than the much cheaper tetracyclines. Moreover, the tetracyclines do not seem to lead to relapses or rapid recurrences. Finally, we must point out that even where the chlamydial infection was probably not adequately treated because penicillins or cephalosporins had been prescibed for patients with acute influenza-like symptoms or even mild pneumonia, the patients treated nevertheless appeared to be cured.

Future developments in the diagnosis and treatment of infections associated with *C. pneumoniae* may lead to a more widespread recognition of the infection and, in turn, to the more accurate use of antimicrobial agents. In particular, new perspec-tives may open up for the prevention of coronary arterial disease.

References

1. Aldous MB, Grayston JT, Wang SP, Foy HM (1992) Seroepidemiology of *Chlamydia pneu-moniae* TWAR infection in Seattle Families, 1966-1979. J Infect Dis 166:646-649
2. Atmar RL, Greenberg SB (1989) Pneumonia caused by *Mycoplasma pneumoniae* and the TWAR agent. Semin Respir Infect 4:19-31
3. Beaty CD, Grayston JT, Wang SP et al (1991) *Chlamydia pneumoniae*, strain TWAR, infec-tion in patients with chronic obstructive pulmonary disease. Am Rev Respir Dis 144:1408-1410
4. Berdal BP, Fields PI, Mitchell SH, Hoddevik G (1990) Isolation of *Chlamydia pneumoniae* during an adenovirus outbreak. In: Chlamydia infections. Bowie WR et al (eds), Cambridge University Press, Cambridge pp 445-448
5. Berdal BP, Scheel O, Øgaard AR, Hoel T, Gutteberg TJ, Ånestad G (1992) Spread of subclin-ical *Chlamydia pneumoniae* infection in a closed community. Scand J Infect Dis 24:431-436
6. Blasi F, Cosentini R, Denti F, Allegra L (1994) *Chlamydia pneumoniae* infection in two unrelated families. Eur Respir J 7:102-4
7. Blasi F, Legnani D, Lombardo VM, Negretto GG, Magliano E, Pozzoli R, Chiodo F, Fasoli A, Allegra L (1993) *Chlamydia pneumoniae* infection in acute exacerbations of COPD. Eur Respir J 6:19-22
8. Bourke SJ (1993) Chlamydial respiratory infections: common but difficult to diagnose. BMJ 306:1219-1220
9. Erntell M, Ljunggren K, Gadd T, Persson K (1989) Erythema nodosum - a manifestation of *Chlamydia pneumoniae* (strain TWAR) infection. Scand J Infect Dis 21:693-696

10. Grayston JT, Kuo CC, Wang SP, Altman J (1986) A new *Chlamydia psittaci* strain, TWAR, isolated in acute respiratory tract infections. N Engl J Med 315:161-168
11. Grayston JT, Campbell LA, Kuo CC, Mordhorst CH, Saikku P, Thom DH (1990) A new respiratory tract pathogen: *Chlamydia pneumoniae* strain TWAR. J Infect Dis 161:618-625
12. Grayston JT (1993) *Chlamydia in atherosclerosis*. Circulation 87:1408-1409
13. Haidl S, Ivarsson S, Bjerre I, Persson K (1992) Guillain Barré Syndrome after *Chlamydia pneumoniae* infection. N Engl J Med 326:576-577
14. Hahn DL (1993) Another possible risk factor for airway disease. Chest 104:649
15. Hammerschlag MR, Qumei KK, Roblin PM (1992) In vitro activities of azithromycin, clarithromycin, L-ofloxacin and other antibiotics against *Chlamydia pneumoniae*. Antimicrob Agents Chemother 36:1573-1574
16. Kleemola M, Saikku P, Viasakorpi R, Wang SP, Grayston JT (1988) Epidemics of pneumonia caused by TWAR, a new *Chlamydia* organism, in military trainees in Finland. J Infect Dis 157:230-236
17. Komaroff AL, Wang SP, Lee J, Grayston JT (1992) No association of chronic *Chlamydia pneumoniae* infection with chronic fatigue syndrome. J Infect Dis 165:184
18. Linnanmäki E, Leinonen M, Mattila K, Nieminen MS, Valtonen V, Saikku P (1993) *Chlamydia pneumoniae* specific circulating immune complexes in patients with chronic coronary heart disease. Circulation 87:1130-1134
19. Marrie TJ, Harczy M, Mann OE, Landymore RW, Raza A, Wang SP, Grayston JT (1990) Culture-negative endocarditis probably due to *Chlamydia pneumoniae*. J Infect Dis 161:127-129
20. Marrie TJ, Grayston JT, Wang SP, Kuo CC (1987) Pneumonia associated with the TWAR strain of *Chlamydia*. Ann Intern Med 106:5007-5011
21. Marrie TJ (1993) *Chlamydia pneumoniae*. Thorax 48:1- 4
22. Maesen FPV, Davies BI, Costongs MAL (1992) Are high serum titres against *Chlamydia pneumoniae* significant in patients with community-acquired pneumonia? Eur Respir J [Suppl 15]:343
23. Mordhorst CH, Wang SP, Grayston JT (1992) Outbreak of *Chlamydia pneumoniae* infection in four farm families. Eur J Clin Microbiol Infect Dis 11:617-620
24. Rumbak MJ, Baselski V, Belenchia JM, Griffin JP (1993) Case report: acute postoperative respiratory failure caused by *Chlamydia pneumoniae* and diagnosed by bronchoalveolar lavage. Am J Med Sci 6:390-393
25. Saikku P, Wang SP, Kleemola M, Brander E, Rusanen E, Grayston JT (1985) An epidemic of mild pneumonia due to an unusual strain of *Chlamydia psittaci*. J Infect Dis 151:832-839
26. Saikku P, Mattila K, Nieminen MS, Huttunen JK, Leinonen M, Ekman MR, Makela PH, Valtona V (1988) Serological evidence of an association of a novel *Chlamydia*, TWAR, with chronic coronary heart disease and acute myocardial infarction. Lancet ii:983-985
27. Saikku P, Ruutu P, Leinonen M, Panelius J, Tupasi TE, Grayston JT (1988) Acute lower respiratory tract infection associated with Chlamydial TWAR antibody in filipino children. J Infect Dis 158:1095-1097
28. Shor A, Kuo CC, Patton DL (1992) Detection of *Chlamydia pneumoniae* in coronary arterial fatty streaks and atheromatous plaques. S Afr Med J 82:158-161
29. Stolk-Engelaar MVM, Peeters MF (1990) Heeft *Chlamydia* TWAR betekenis in Nederland ? Ned Tijdschr Geneeskd 134:1094-1097
30. Sundelöf B, Gnarpe H, Gnarpe J (1993) An unusual manifestation of *Chlamydia pneumoniae* infection: meningitis, hepatitis, iritis and atypical erythema nodosum. Scand J Infect Dis 25:259-261
31. Thom DH, Grayston JT (1991) Infections with *Chlamydia pneumoniae* strain TWAR. Clin Chest Med 12:245-256

32. Thom DH, Grayston JT, Siscovick DS, Wang SP, Weiss NS, Daling JR (1992) Association of prior infection with *Chlamydia pneumoniae* and angiographically demonstrated coronary artery disease. JAMA 268:68-72
33. Torres A, El-Ebiary M (1993) Relevance of *Chlamydia pneumoniae* in community-acquired respiratory infections. Eur Respir J 6:7-8
34. Van den Abeele AM, Van Renterghem L, Willems K, Plum J (1992) Prevalence of antibodies to *Chlamydia pneumoniae* in a Belgian population. J Infect 25 [Suppl 1]:87-90
35. Wesslen L, Pahlson C, Friman G, Fohlman J, Lindquist O, Johansson C (1992) Myocarditis caused by *Chlamydia pneumoniae* (TWAR) and sudden unexpected death in a Swedish elite orienteer. Lancet 340:427-428

Chapter 7 Immunology of *Chlamydia pneumoniae*

MAIJA LEINONEN, AINO LAURILA, KIRSI LAITINEN AND HELJÄ M. SURCEL

Introduction

All *chlamydia* are obligate intracellular parasites and at their simplest can be regarded as highly specialized gram-negative bacteria with two developmental forms: infective elementary bodies and reproductive reticulate bodies. Both the structural components of the chlamydial cell (virulence factors) and the host cell factors - how the host resists to chlamydial infection - play a role in the immunological mechanisms associated with chlamydial infections. To date very little is known about the immunology of *C. pneumoniae*, but evidently most immunological mechanisms associated with other chlamydial infections are also involved in *C. pneumoniae* infections.

Different chlamydial species and even biovars infect different cell types (Table 1). Most *C. trachomatis* biovars infect mucosal epithelium and tend to remain localized or to spread along mucosal epithelium (e.g. in trachoma and pelvic inflammatory disease). However, *C. psittaci* and the lymphogranuloma venereum biovar (LGV) of *C. trachomatis* are able to cause infections in a variety of cell types including mononuclear phagocytes. It has recently been shown that *C. pneumoniae* also exhibits the capacity of multiplying within alveolar macrophages [1], human monocytes and vascular endothelial cells [2]. Monocytes and macrophages are important cells in the immunological defence mechanisms and the survival and multiplication of *C. pneumoniae* inside these cells may confer the immunological features of *C. pneumoniae* infections. Furthermore, when *C. pneumoniae* is residing in alveolar macrophages and especially in vascular endothelial cells, bacteria and their structural components - either shed from infected cells or liberated when host cells are destroyed - have an easy access to circulation. These components can bind to antibodies present in circulation forming immune complexes which maintain inflammatory reactions in the vascular system.

Table 1. Host cell tropism of Chlamydial species

Species, Biovar	Host cell
C. trachomatis	epithelial cells
C. trachomatis, LGV	variety of cell types monocytes, macrophages
C. psittaci	variety of cell types monocytes, macrophages
C. peumoniae	variety of cell types monocytes, macrophages, endothelial cells

All chlamydial species have a tendency to cause chronic infections. Persistent *C. psittaci* infections in birds and mammals have been known for years and infections caused by LGV and *C. psittaci* may persist in humans for 10 to 20 years. Generally most mild acute infections caused by *C. trachomatis* resolve without sequelae, but they can also progress not only to severe chronic inflammation leading to blindness (trachoma) even 50 years after primary infection, but also to infertility, ectopic pregnancies and reactive arthritis. *C. pneumoniae* is evidently capable of causing chronic infections and it has already been associated with several chronic conditions, including chronic bronchitis [3, 4], adult onset asthma [4, 5], sarcoidosis [6, 7] and chronic coronary heart disease [8-10]. The immunopathological mechanisms leading to different chronic conditions are not known at present.

Antibody Response to *C. pneumoniae* Infections

Being gram-negative bacteria, *Chlamydia* have a typical cell wall component, lipopolysaccharide (LPS). The chemical compositions of LPSs from both *C. trachomatis* [11] and *C. psittaci* [12] have been described, and they contain typical components of gram-negative LPS. Chlamydial LPS is of a deep-rough type having only an acidic ketodeoxioctonate (KDO) trisaccharide-unit linked to the lipid A part of the molecule. The endotoxin activity of chlamydial LPS seems to be much lower than that of gram-negative bacteria [12]. The decreased toxicity might be an advantage to *chlamydia*. It is shed from infected cells and high endotoxin activity could thus immediately lead to a deleteriuos response in the host.

Furthermore, as in the case of *C. pneumoniae*, infected alveolar macrophages or endothelial cells are in close contact with the circulation. By demonstrating the presence of chlamydial LPS containing immune complexes in diseases associated with possible chronic chlamydial infections like acute myocardial infarction and chronic coronary heart disease [9,13,14] we have confirmed that chlamydial LPS undoubtedly has an access to circulation. However, shock-like symptoms have never been described in connection with chlamydial infections.

The outer membrane proteins (OMP) of *C. pneumoniae* seem to be somewhat different from those of other chlamydial species. The major outer membrane protein, MOMP, of *C. trachomatis* is highly immunogenic and is also responsible for serotype-specificity. The MOMP of *C. pneumoniae* seems to be only poorly immunogenic and so far no differences in the amino acid sequences of MOMPs from different *C. pneumoniae* isolates have been found [15]. The cysteine-rich 60 kDa protein, OMP2, is possibly very conservative as well (Rasmussen S, personal communication). When antibody responses to different isolates of *C. pneumoniae* are compared, the kinetics of responses seeem to be different suggesting that there are different immunotypes among *C. pneumoniae* strains (16, our unpublished data). However, at the moment we do not know the structural components which may confer serotype specificity of *C. pneumoniae*.

Heat shock (or stress) proteins have important functions in cellular matabolism and they aid cells in dealing with environmental stimuli [17]. They are highly conserved and exhibit wide cross-reactivity among eucaryotic cells, parasites and bacteria [18,19]. During acute and chronic infections caused by parasites and bacteria, antibodies to heat shock proteins are produced and these may act as "autoimmune" antibodies and lead to tissue injury. Recent studies have shown that *Chlamydia* possess at least two heat shock proteins, a 57 kD protein belonging to the 60 hsp family and a 70 kD protein belonging to the 70 hsp family [20-22].

Serum antibody response to surface structures of *C. pneumoniae* can be demonstrated by the micro-immunofluorescence method during acute infections. Primary infections are characterized by a rapid IgM response and delayed IgG responses, which can be documented as late as 6 weeks after the onset of disease [23, 24]. However, it is possible that the delayed response may simply be due to the fact that the antigens used by most laboratories are two original *C. pneumoniae* strains, TW 183 and IOL 207, and not the strains circulating in the population being tested. In reinfections no IgM antibodies are found and both IgG and IgA responses are more rapid than in primary infections [24, 25]. Complement fixing chlamydial group-specific antibodies are formed in primary infections especially in young adults, but they are not generally seen in reinfections [25, 26]. However, patients with both primary infection and reinfection show an antibody response towards the lipopolysaccharide, when measured by enzyme immunoassay [25].

Immunoblotting analyses of the sera from infected humans have shown that antibody responses are directed against several structural proteins, most of them being species-specific [16, 27-29]. In contrast to other chlamydial species, antibody responses to MOMP are only seldom seen. Sera from patients with *C. pneumoniae* infection in the USA have been reported to contain antibodies most frequently towards a high molecular weight 98 kDa protein which has been considered *C. pneumoniae* specific [27], while in chronic infections antibodies frequently recognise 43 kDa and 52 kDa proteins [30]. Two of these proteins, the 98 kDa and 43 kDa proteins, are also recognized by immune complex-bound antibodies in the sera of Finnish patients with chronic coronary heart disease [14]. On the contrary, in a German study, only 14 % of the acute sera reacted with the 98 kDa protein whereas another species-specific 54 kDa protein was recognized by 93 % of the sera containing *C. pneumoniae* antibodies [28]. The great variation in the prevalences of antibodies against different proteins cannot possibly be explained by individual responsiveness to different antigens but rather with epidemic and regional variations of *C. pneumoniae* strains. Protein analyses of several *C. pneumoniae* isolates have proved that quantitative differences can be detected in the relative amounts of structural proteins [29].

Antibody prevalence and antibody titers to *C. pneumoniae* increase with age and are at their highest in elderly populations all over the world. Since antibodies are lost after acute infections, the steadily rising titers and prevalences suggest that reinfections and chronic infections are common and that serum antibodies do not protect from these infections. Antibody prevalence to *C. pneumoniae* increases with age, averaging 50% in middle-aged adults [31-33] throughout the world. In the northern sparsely populated areas [34-36] like in Finland and in other Scandinavian countries, *C. pneumoniae* causes widespread epidemics every five to seven years during which young adults and military recruits are particularly affected.

It is possible that after an epidemic the antibody prevalence and antibody titers decrease and when population immunity is sufficiently low and a sufficient number of susceptible young people is available, the new epidemic starts. The antibody prevalence in males is higher than in females and the most striking differences are seen in the oldest age groups. We have also tested *C. pneumoniae* antibodies in an elderly population of a rural community in Finland and both the antibody prevalence and the geometric mean antibody titers resulted higher in males than in females and increased with age suggesting that males are more susceptible to *C. pneumoniae* infections than females [33, 37]. Since antibodies are lost after an acute infection [38] and the prevalence rises steadily, it can be estimated that the majority of people have two or three *C. pneumoniae* infections during their lifetime and evidently primary infection does not protect from reinfections.

Cell-Mediated Immune Response to *C. pneumoniae*

T-cell mediated immunity is considered to be important in the defence against intracellular pathogens such as *Mycobacterium tuberculosis*. Since *Chlamydia* are obligate intracellular parasites it has been suggested that T-cell mediated immunological mechanisms play a role both in the protective and in the destructive immunopathological processes associated with chlamydial infections. In *C. trachomatis* infections, cell mediated immunity is thought to be responsible for chronic scarring processes causing trachoma and tubal obstruction. Interesting data have been obtained concerning a 57 kD protein. As far back as 1962, during trachoma vaccination trials both in humans and in primates, Grayston et al. [39] suggested that immunological mechanisms play a role in the pathogenesis of this disease. The studies showed that prior immunization with killed *chlamydia* actually led to a more severe disease during reinfection suggesting that immunization primed the host for a deleterious hypersensitivity response [40, 41]. In addition, they showed that the disease was even more severe if different *C. trachomatis* serovars were used for the challenge, suggesting that this hypersensitivity response is due to antigens common to the *chlamydia* genus. The most direct evidence of the hypersensitivity reaction has been obtained from experiments in which crude extracts of *chlamydia* elicit severe ocular inflammation in immune animals. In immunized guinea pigs an ocular inflammatory response with histopathological aspects similar to those seen in trachoma or in *chlamydia*-induced infertility can be obtained with chlamydial extracts [42, 43]. The hypersensitivity has been shown to be closely associated with a 57 kD protein [44]. In addition to the pathological role of the 57 kD protein in ocular infection, there are reports that women affected by salpingitis, both with and without infertility, have different reaction patterns to this protein [45] suggesting that similar pathogenetic mechanisms may also play a role in infertility caused by *C. trachomatis*.

The hypothesis concerning the role of heat shock proteins in the pathogenesis of chlamydial infections, first suggested by Morrison et al. [46] and Bavoil et al. [47], is the following: chlamydial infections are usually limited anatomically and temporally by potent cell mediated and humoral immune responses. After the primary infection, hypersensitivity reactions with tissue injury can occur upon re-exposure to the organism, such as in trachoma. During this phase organisms are rarely isolated, but inflammatory symptoms are strong. Recent data on the role of mycobacterial stress proteins and auto-reactive T-lymphocytes suggest autoimmune mechanisms in the pathogenesis of chronic mycobacterial disease. These mechanisms might also play a role in the immunopathologic sequelae of chronic chlamydial infections.

The role of T-lymphocytes in protective immunity against *C. trachomatis* is not known. However, in the guinea pig animal model both humoral and cell mediated immunity seem to be required for the overcoming of the disease, and in mice CD4+ T-cells have been shown to have an important role in cell mediated defence mechanisms [48]. T-cell mediated immunity against *C. pneumoniae* has thus far been studied in persons who have acquired laboratory infection caused by *C. pneumoniae* strain Kajaani 6 [49]. A definite antigen-specific lymphocyte proliferation response, which started to increase at 3 weeks and had a peak value at 8 to 9 weeks after the onset of symptoms, was recorded. As shown in Figure 1, T-cell responses to *C. pneumoniae* antigens are significantly stronger in healthy, seropositive individuals than in seronegative persons. In contrast to healthy individuals in whom the T-cell reactivity is specific to *C. pneumoniae* antigens, we have recently observed that patients with severe coronary heart disease elicit a T-cell response that is cross-reactive with different chlamydial species and which might be directed against conservative protein epitopes in MOMP or even against chlamydial heat shock proteins shared by different chlamydial species. Moreover, high antibody titers to *C. pneumoniae* in patients with coronary heart disease were often associated with a decreased T-cell reactivity against *C. pneumoniae*. These preliminary results suggest that T-cell immunity might be important in the protection against *C. pneumoniae*, and that in chronic infections or in reinfections T-cells may also be responsible for the immunopathological processes associated with the disease (Surcel et al., to be published).

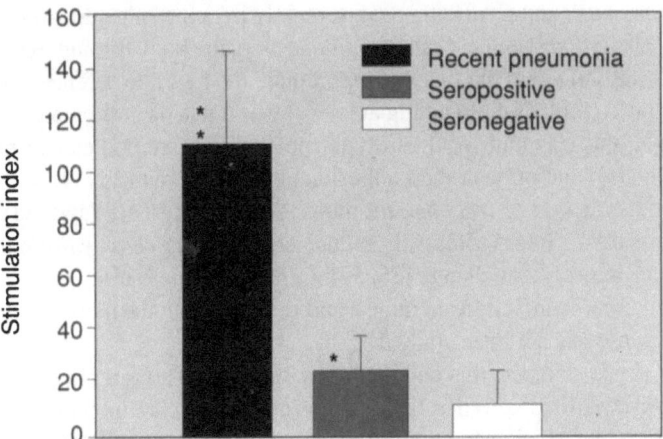

Fig. 1. Lymphocyte proliferative responses (stimulation index) to *C. pneumoniae* antigen. *C. pneumoniae* specific antibody titers were ≥ 64 in subjects with acute pneumonia, > 32 in seropositive subjects and ≤ 8 in seronegative subjects. Proliferative responses were compared with t-test. *$p<0.03$, **$p<0.01$

The role of cytokines in the cellular resistance to chlamydial infections has been quite intensively studied in recent years. It has been shown that interferon-γ (IFNγ), interleukin-1 (IL1), interleukin-6 (IL6) and tumor necrosis factor-a (TNFα) are produced in chlamydial infections and they also confer resistance to infection [50, 51]. Previous studies have also suggested that small concentrations of IFNγ may lead to a persistent *C. trachomatis* infection in cell cultures. However, cytokines also partecipate in inflammatory reactions, and it has been indicated that several reactions associated with endotoxin shock can be induced by replacing LPS with TNF. Furthermore it has recently been shown that TNF inhibits lipoprotein lipase, leading to mobilization of lipids and to increased serum triglyceride and lowered HDL levels [53]. We have previously shown that *C. pneumoniae* is capable of inducing IL1 and TNF production in human monocytes [54]. We have also shown that in acute *C. pneumoniae* pneumonia, triglyceride levels are significantly higher and HDL levels, particularly HDL2, significantly lower than in either viral or pneumococcal pneumonias (Leinonen et al. to be published). It can be speculated that in chronic *C. pneumoniae* infections the continuous production of TNF might lead to a serum lipid pattern similar to that which is considered as a risk factor for coronary heart disease.

Immunological Protection from *C. pneumoniae* Infection in the Mouse Model

With the advance in chlamydial molecular biology, animal models have became important in understanding the immunopathology of human chlamydial disease and they provide an obvious mean for analyzing immunity to precisely defined chlamydial components associated with both protective and pathological immune mechanisms.

Current knowledge on experimental *chlamydial* infections is based on research using *C. trachomatis* and *C. psittaci* strains, mainly in guinea pig and mouse models. Like other chlamydial species, *C. pneumoniae* enters the body through mucosal surfaces. Local antibodies are likely to be important in the first line defence, with serum antibodies and T-cell immunity acting at later stage. It has been shown that circulating IgM, IgA and IgG and local serotype-specific IgA antibodies can neutralize chlamydia *in vitro* and prevent their adhesion and/or endocytosis [54, 55]. Furthermore, antibodies against *C. trachomatis*, mouse pneumonitis agent and LGV strains, given intranasally or intraperitoneally reduce significantly *chlamydial* numbers in the lungs after intranasal challenge [56, 57]. *C. pneumoniae* is also capable of causing acute and chronic infections in mouse and monkeys, but the nature of protective immune response has not been studied.

Several studies indicate that cell mediated immune responses play an important role in chlamydial disease. When thymusless (nude mice) are infected with mouse pneumonitis agent they develop a more serious disease than control mice [58, 59]. Nude mice recover from infection if they receive antigen specific T-cell lines [60]. The importance of cell-mediated immunity was also emphasized in a study where no difference was observed between mice having B-cell deficiency or normal mice during genital infection or when resistance to reinfection was evaluated [61]. In a mouse genital infection model it has also been shown that antigen-specific T-cells are needed in the mucosal surfaces of the genital tract in order to prevent reinfection by *C. trachomatis* [62]. The role of CD8+ T-cells in chlamydial immunopathology has not yet been proved.

Mice provide a good animal model to study chlamydial infections. The availability of immunologically defined inbred mouse strains and specific reagents allows statistically adequate studies on the immunopathology of chlamydial infections. Mouse models to study immunopathogenesis and defence mechanism in *C. pneumoniae* infection have been developed [63, 64]. Both these studies have shown that there is a strong antibody response against *C. pneumoniae* peaking at 3 to 4 weeks after intranasal challenge. *C. pneumoniae* can be isolated from lung tissues for more than two weeks and there is an inverse relationship between isolation yield and specific antibody levels.

In the model of Yang et al. [63] primary infection induced an acute, patchy pneumonia with polymorphonuclear leukocytes and exudate in lung alveoli and bronchi that in two weeks turned to a predominantly monocytic infiltration. In our model [65], using ten times lower inoculum of the bacteria - which probably is clinically more relevant dose - no purulent pneumonia was seen. Histology showed bronchopneumonia that was characterized by a chronic type of inflammation with perivascular and peribronchial lymphocyte infiltrations and minor interstitial inflammation (Fig. 2B). The changes developed more slowly than in the Yang's model, but were as

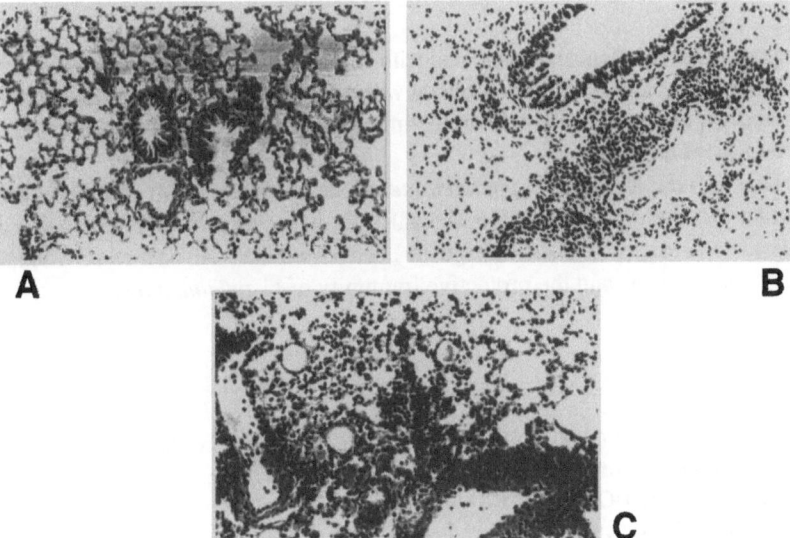

Fig. 2. Histopathological findings of the lung in *C. pneumoniae* infection. **A.** Three days after the bacterial challenge the lung is still normal. **B.** Two weeks later peribronchial and perivascular lymphocyte and plasmacyte infiltrations spread to interstitium, but no purulent inflammation is found. **C.** When the bacterial challenge is given together with anti-*C. pneumoniae* immune serum, an acute inflammation with polymorphonuclear leukocytes is induced already on the sixth day after challenge (original magnification x200)

long-lasting and stayed demonstrable for several weeks after the challenge. Our recent data [65] on the reinfections in the mice indicate that bacterial cultures are positive only for a couple of days after the rechallenge. However, the inflammatory changes in the lungs are as strong and long-lasting and develop earlier than the changes seen in primary infection. When convalescent or hyperimmune serum is given intraperitoneally prior the intranasal challenge, chlamydia cultures stay negative, but the lung histology shows acute pneumonia with polymorphonuclear leukocytes (Fig. 2C).

After *C. pneumoniae* infection, *chlamydia* may remain in the body in the latent state during which it can be reactivated by immunosuppression. By using the study protocol described by Yang et al. [66] for *C. trachomatis*, we have shown that when mice were treated with cortisone after recovery from primary infection, i.e. at the time when no chlamydia could be any more found by culture from the lungs, *C. pneumoniae* could be reisolated from lung tissue two weeks after the cortisone treatment was started (K. Laitinen, unpublished data).

The results from animal studies suggest that antibodies, i.e. humoral immunity, may contribute to the protection and that the strong inflammatory response seen in the lungs after the rechallenge of mice with *C. pneumoniae* may be due to the immunodestructive action of T- cell mediated immunity.

Summary

Immunological mechanisms associated with *C. pneumoniae* infections are still largely unknown. Chronic infections associated with *C. pneumoniae* seem to be very common and we do not know at present the immunological mechanisms leading to different clinical pictures.

The high incidence of *C. pneumoniae* infections suggested by high prevalence of antibodies in elderly population, as well as the association of *C. pneumoniae* with severe chronic sequelae, make emerge the need for studies both on the immunopathogenetic mechanisms and the protective immunity of *C. pneumoniae*.

References

1. Black CM, Perez R (1990) *Chlamydia pneumoniae* multiplies within pulmonary macrophages. In: Abstr 90th Annual Meet A.S.M., Anaheim,1990; abstr D-1, Amer Soc Microbiol, Washington DC, 82
2. Kaukoranta-Tolvanen SS, Saikku P, Leinonen M (1992) Growth of *Chlamydia pneumoniae* in endothelial cells compared to other cell types Proc European Soc for Chlamydia Res 2:168
3. Blasi F, Legnani D, Lombardo VM, Negretto GG, Magliano E, Pozzoli R, Chiodo F, Fasoli A, Allegra L (1993) *Chlamydia pneumoniae* infection in acute exacerbations of COPD. Eur Respir J 6:19-22
4. von Herzen L, Leinonen M, Koskinen R, Liippo K, Saikku P (1994) Evidence of persistent *Chlamydia pneumoniae* infection in patients with chronic obstructive pulmonary dis-

Immunology of *Chlamydia pneumoniae* 47

ease. In: Proceedings of the 8th International Symposium on Human Chlamydial infections, Chantilly 19-24 June 1994, Orfila J et al (eds), Esculapio Bologna, pp 473-476
5. Hahn DL, Dodge RW, Golubjatnikov R (1991) Association of *Chlamydia pneumoniae* (strain TWAR) infection with wheezing, asthmatic bronchitis, and adult-onset asthma. JAMA 266:225-230
6. Grönhagen-Riska C, Saikku P, Riska H, Fröseth B, Grayston JT (1988) Antibodies to TWAR - a novel Type of *Chlamydia* - in sarcoidosis. In: Sarcoidosis and other granulomatous disorders. Grassi C et al (eds), Elsevier Scientific Publ, Amsterdam, pp 297-301
7. Black CM, Bullard JC, Staton GW, Hutwagner LC, Perez RL (1992) Seroprevalence of *Chlamydia pneumoniae* antibodies in patients with pulmonary sarcoidosis in North Central Georgia. Proc European Soc for Chlamydia Res 2:175
8. Saikku P, Mattila K, Nieminen MS, Huttunen JK, Leinonen M, Ekman MR, Mäkelä PH, Valtonen V (1988) Serological evidence of an association of a novel *Chlamydia*, TWAR, with chronic heart disease and acute myocardial infarction. Lancet ii:983-985
9. Saikku P, Leinonen M, Tenkanen L, Ekman MR, Linnanmärki E, Manninen V, Mänttäri M, Frick MM, Huttunen JK (1992) Chronic *Chlamydia pneumoniae* infection as a risk factor for coronary heart disease in the Helsinki Heart Study. Ann Int Med 116:273-278
10. Kuo CC, Shor A, Campbell LA, Fukushi H, Patton DL, Grayston JT (1993) Demonstration of *Chlamydia pneumoniae* in atherosclerotic lesions of coronary arteries. J Infect Dis 167:845-849
11. Nurminen M; Rietschel ET, Brade H (1985) Chemical characterization of *Chlamydia trachomatis* lipopolysaccaride. Infect Immun 48:573-575
12. Brade L, Schramek S, Schade U, Brade H (1986) Chemical, biological and immunochemical properties of *Chlamydia psittaci* lipopolysaccharide. Infec Immun 54:567-574
13. Leinonen M, Linnanmäki E, Mattila K, Nieminen MS, Leirisalo-Repo M, Valtonen V, Saikku P (1990) Circulating immune complexes containing Chlamydial lypopolisaccharide in acute myocardial infarction. Microbial Patoghenesis 9:67-73
14. Linnanmärki E, Leinonen M, Ekman MR, Mattila K, Nieminen MS, Valtonen V, Saikkui P (1993) *Chlamydia pneumoniae* specific circulating immune complexes in chronic heart disease. Circulation 87:1130-1134
15. Gaydos CA, Quinn TC, Bobo LD, Eiden JJ (1992) Similarity of *Chlamydia pneumoniae* strains in the variable domain IV region of the major outer membrane protein gene. Infect Immun 60:5319-5323
16. Black CM, Johnson JE, Farshy CE, Brown TM, Berdal BP (1991) Antigenic variation among strains of *Chlamydia pneumoniae*. J Clin Microbiol 29:1312-1316
17. Lindquist S, Craig EA (1988) The heat shock proteins. Ann Rev Genet 22:631-677
18. Young DB, Ivanyi J, Cox JH, Lamb JR (1987) The 65 kDa antigen of mycobacteria-a common bacterial protein. Immunol Today 8:215-219
19. Young D, Lathigra R, Hendrix R, Sweetser R, Young RA (1988) Stress proteins are immune targets in leprosy and tuberculosis. Proc Natl Acad Sci 85:4267-4270
20. Menozzi FD, Menozzi-Dejaiffe C, Nano FE (1989) Molecular cloning of a gene encoding a *Chlamydia psittaci* 57 kDa protein that shares antigenic determinants with ca. 60 kDa proteins present in many gram-negative bacteria. FEBS Letters 58:59-64
21. Cerrone MC, Ma JJ, Stephens RS (1991) Cloning and sequence of the gene for heat shock protein 60 from *Chlamydia trachomatis* and immunological reactivity of the protein. Infect Immun 59:79-90
22. Birkelund S, Lundemose AG, Christiansen G (1990) The 75 kDa cytoplasmatioc *Chlamydia trachomatis* L"2 polypeptide is a DNA-like protein. Infect Immun 58:2098-2104
23. Grayston JT, Campbell LA, Kuo CC, Mordhorst CH, Saikku P, Thom DH, Wang SP

(1990) A new respiratory tract pathogen, *Chlamydia pneumoniae* strain TWAR. J Infect Dis 161:618-625

24. Ekman MR, Grayston JT, Visakorpi R, Kleemola M, Kuo CC, Saikku P (1993) An epidemic of infections due to *Chlamydia pneumoniae* in military conscripts. Clin Infect Dis 17:420-425

25. Ekman MR, Leinonen M, Syrjälä H, Linnanmäki E, Kujala P, Saikku P (1993) Evaluation of serological methods in the diagnosis of *Chlamydia pneumoniae* during an epidemic in Finland. Eur J Clin Microbiol 12:756-760

26. Marrie TJ, Grayston JT, Kuo CC (1987) Pneumonia associated with TWAR strain of *Chlamydia*. Ann Int Med 106:507-511

27. Campbell LA, Kuo CC, Wang SP, Grayston JT (1990) Serological response to *Chlamydia pneumoniae* infection. J Clin Microbiol 28:1261-1264

28. Freidank HM, Herr AS, Jacobs E (1993) Identifications of *Chlamydia pneumoniae* specific protein antigens in immunoblots. Eur J Clin Microbiol Infect Dis 112:947-951

29. Iijima Y, Miyashita N, Kishimoto T, Kanamoto Y, Soejima R, Matsumoto A (1994) Characterization of *Chlamydia pneumoniae* species specific proteins immunodominant in humans. J Clin Microbiol 32:583-588

30. Puolakkainen M, Kuo CC, Shor A, Wang SP, Grayston JT, Campbell LA (1993) Serological response to *Chlamydia pneumoniae* in adults with coronary arterial fatty streaks and fibrolipid plaques. J Clin Microbiol 31:2212-2214

31. Forsey T, Darougar S, Treharne JD, Jones BR, Herring J (1986) Prevalence in human beings of antibodies to *Chlamydia* IOL-207, an atypical strain of Chlamydia. J Infect 12:145-152

32. Wang SP, Grayston JT (1990) Population prevalence antibody to *Chlamydia pneumoniae*, strain TWAR. In: Proceedings of the 7th International Symposium on Human Chlamydial Infections, Bowie WR et al (eds) pp 402-405

33. Saikku P (1992) The epidemiology and significance of *Chlamydia pneumoniae*. J Infect 25 (S1):27-34

34. Bruu AL, Aasen S, Tjaland S, Birkeland S, Flugsrud L (1984) An outbreak of ornithosis in Norway in 1981. Scand J Infect Dis 16:145-152

35. Grayston JT, Mordhorst CH, Bruu AL, Vene S, Wang SP (1989) Countrywide epoidemics of *Chlamydia pneumoniae*, strain TWAR, in Scandinavia, 1981-1983. J Infect Dis 159:1111-1114

36. Kleemola M, Saikku P, Viasakorpi R, Wang SP, Grayston JT (1988) Epidemics of pneumonia caused by TWAR, a new *Chlamydia* organism, in military trainees in Finland. J Infect Dis 157:230-236

37. Töyrylä M, Isoaho R, Puolijoki H, Huhti E, Kivelä SL, Saikku P (1992) Prevalence of *Chlamydia pneumoniae* antibodies of enderly population in Finnish rural district. Proc European Soc for Chlamydia Res 2:293

38. Patnode D, Wang SP, Grayston JT (1990) Persistence of *Chlamydia pneumoniae*, strain TWAR, microimmunofluorescent antibody. In : Proceedings of the 7th International Symposium on Human Chlamydial Infections, Bowie WR et al (eds) pp 406-409

39. Grayston JT, Woolridge RL, Wang SP (1962) Trachoma vaccine studies on Taiwan. Ann N.Y. Acad Sci 98:352-367

40. Grayston JT, Wang SP, Yreh LJ, Kuo CC (1985) Importance of reinfection in the pathogenesis of trachoma. Rev Inf Dis 7:717-725

41. Wang SP, Grayston JT, Alexander ER (1967) Trachoma vaccine studies in monkeys. Am J Ophtalmol 63:1615-1630

42. Watkins NG, Hadlow WJ, Moos AB, Caldwell HD (1986) Ocular delayed bypersensitiv-

ity: apathogenetic mechanism of Chlamydial conjunctivitis in guinea pig. Proc Natl Acad Sci 83:7480-7487
43. Moller BR, Weström L, Ahrons S, Ripa T, Swensson L, Mecklelburg C, Henrikson H, Märdh Pa (1979) *Chlamydia trachomatis* infection of the fallopian tubes. Br J Vener Dis 55:422-429
44. Morrison RP, Belland RJ, Lyng K, Calwell HD (1989) Chlamydial hypersensitivity antigen is a stress response protein. J Exp Med 170:1271-1283
45. Brunham RC, Peeling R, Maclean I, McDowell J, Persson K, Osser S (1987) Postabortal *Chlamydia trachomatis* salpingitis: correlating risk with antigen-specific serological responses and with neutralization. J Infect Dis 155:749-755
46. Morrison RP (1990) Chlamydial 57 kDa stress response protein is deleterious immune target. In: Microbial determinants of virulence and host response. Ayuoub EM et al (eds) American Society of Microbiology, Washington DC, 243-250
47. Bavoil P, Stephens RS, Falkow S (1990) A soluble 60 kDa antigen of *Chlamydia spp.* is homologue of Escherichia coli GroEl. Molec Microbiol 4:461-469
48. Rank RGL, Soderberg LSF, Sanders MM, Batteiger B (1989) Role of cell mediated immunity in the resolution of secondary Chlamydial genital infection in guinea pigs infected with the agent of guinea pig inclusion conjunctivitis. Infect Immun 57:706-710
49. Surcel HM, Syrjälä H, Leinonen M, Saikku P, Herva E (1993) Cell-mediated immunity to *Chlamydia pneumoniae* measured as lymphocytes blast transformation in vitro. Infect Immun 61:2196-2199
50. Holtman H, Shemer-Avni Y, Wessel K, Sarov I, Wallach D (1990) Inhibition of growth of *Chlamydia trachomatis* by tumor necrosis factor is accompanied by increased prostaglandin synthesis. Infect Immun 58:3168-3172
51. Williams DM, Magee DM, Bonewald LF, Smith JG, Bleicker CA, Byrne GI, Schacter J (1990) A role in vivo for tumor necrosis factor alpha in host defence against *Chlamydia trachomatis*. Infect Immun 58:1572-1576
52. Kawakami M, Pekala PH, Lance MD, Cerami A (1983) Lipoprotein lipase supression in 3T3 L1 cells by an induced mediator from exudate cells. Proc Natl Acad Sci 79:912-916
53. Kaukoranta-Tolvanen SS, Teppo AM, Leinonen M, Saikku P, Laitinen K (1992) *Chlamydia pneumoniae* induces the production of TNFα, IL-1b, and IL-6 by human monocytes. Proc European Soc for Chlamydia Res 2:85
54. Howard LV (1975) Neutralization of *Chlamydia trachomatis* in cell culture. Infect Immun 11: 698-703
55. Ainsworth S, Allan I, Pearce JH (1979) Differential neutralization of spontaneous and centrifuge assisted Chlamydial activity. J Gen Microbiol 114:61-67
56. Williams DM, Schacter J, Coalson J, Grubbs B (1984) Cellular immunity to the mouse pneumonitis agent. J Infect Dis 149:630-639
57. Cui ZD, LaScolea LJ, Fischer J, Ogra PL (1989) Immunoprophylaxis of *Chlamydia trachomatis* lymphogranuloma venereum pneumonitis in mice by oral immunizations. Infect Immun 57:739-744
58. Williams DM, Schacter J, Drutz DJ, Sumaya CV (1981) Pneumonia due to *Chlamydia trachomatis* in the immunocompromized (nude) mouse. J Infect Dis 143:238-241
59. Rank RG, Soderberg LS, Barron Al (1985) Chronic Chlamydial infection in congenitally athymic mice. Infect Immun 48:847-849
60. Ramsey KH, Rank RG (1991) Resolution of Chlamydial genital infection with antigen specific T-lymphocyte lines. Infect Immun 59:925-931
61. Romagnani S (1992) Induction of TH1 and TH2 responses: a key role for the natural immune response. Immunology Today 13:379-381

62. Igiewtseme JU, Rank RG (1991) Susceptibility to reinfection after a primary Chlamydial genital infection is associated with a decrease of antigen specific T -cells in the genital tract. Infect Immun 59:1346-1351
63. Yang ZP, Kuo CC, Grayston JT (1993) A mouse model of *Chlamydia pneumoniae* strain TWAR pneumonitis. Infect Immun 61:2037-2040
64. Kaukoranta-Tolvanen SS, Laurila Al, Saikku P, Leinonen M, Liesirova L, Laitinen K (1993) Experimental infection of *Chlamydia pneumoniae* in mice. Microbial Pathogenesis 15:293-302
65. Laitinen K, Laurila A, Leinonen M, Saikku P (1994) Experimental *Chlamydia pneumoniae* infection in mice: effect of reinfection and passive protection by immune serum. In: Proceedings of the 8th International Symposium on Human Chlamydial infections, Chantilly 19-24 June 1994, Orfila J et al (eds) Esculapio, Bologna, pp 545-548
66. Yang YS, Kuo CC, Chen WJ (1983) Reactivation of *Chlamydia trachomatis* lung infection in mice by cortisone. Infect Immun 39:655-658

Chapter 8   Chronic *Chlamydia pneumoniae* Infections

Pekka Saikku

Introduction

Chronic infections are the most important form of chlamydial infections. Moreover, as the average lifetime increases the importance of chronic infections and associated late sequalae also rises. In *C. trachomatis* infections it can take decades before blindness develops in trachoma, important symptoms of lymphogranuloma venereum (LGV) are only seen after years of disease progression, and an episode of male non-gonococcal urethritis may sometimes suggest a woman in danger of developing ectopic pregnancy and infertility due to a chronic silent pelvic inflammatory disease (PID) [48]. The discovery of *C. pneumoniae*, an extremely common *Chlamydia* which readily invades the lung, prompted a study on the possibility of a chronic involvement of this organ. Through the lungs a pathogen has an easy opportunity for further dissemination inside the body, and *C. pneumoniae* has also been associated with non respiratory chronic diseases.

Diagnosis

Although diagnosis of acute *C. pneumoniae* infection is difficult, there is an even greater problem in diagnosing the chronic diseases it might cause. The amount of infective agent in acute *C. pneumoniae* infections seems to be quite low in most cases, and it could be still lower in chronic infections. The most difficult diagnostic problem lies in the possibility of a "hit and run" situation, where the agent has triggered an abnormal reaction, a self-supporting process causing progression of the disease, although the inducer has disappeared.

Culture

It is a well known phenomenon in *C. trachomatis* studies that in chronic infections chlamydial culture is rarely positive, although in acute infections the agent is relatively easy to cultivate [14, 62, 64]. This is understandable since in chronic infections the lesion is loaded with activated defence mechanisms. In the isolation procedures, cells which previously protected *C. pneumoniae* are crushed, thus freeing the agent which then makes a vulnerable target for neutralisation. *C. pneumoniae* is generally difficult to isolate even in acute disease conditions; thus a negative result in an isolation test is not a definitive proof where a chronic infection is suspected.

Serology

The first evidence that *C. pneumoniae* might cause chronic conditions was suggested by serology. Studies on antibody prevalences in industrialized countries have shown that in the general population, among different chlamydial species, antibodies against *C. pneumoniae* are by far the most common and the highest titered ones [73]. *C. pneumoniae* titer levels seen with micro-immunofluorescence testing are often comparable to *C. trachomatis* titers occuring in infertile women with chronic PID, or in members of both sexes affected by LGV [72, 73]. These titer levels can be partly explained by a booster effect due to reinfections, but may also suggest infections analogous to chronic deep-sited *C. trachomatis* infections.

Serology is a sentinel test, showing that *C. pneumoniae* infections do not behave in general like *C. trachomatis* infections and points to the possibility of commonly occuring chronic, generalized infections. Serology is however a poor indicator of chronic infection. First, it gives no indication of the site of a possible chronic process; secondly, *C. pneumoniae* antibodies are so common, especially in older age groups, that proving an association with a specific disease is difficult; thirdly, epidemics can temporarily induce high antibody titers in control populations.

Despite these limitations a continuously elevated antibody titer can be not only a sign of a possible chronic infection, but also a sign of a failure in the defence mechanisms battling against an intracellular pathogen. In these circumstances the activation of cell-mediated immunity can therefore become crucial. IgA antibodies seem to be more reliable markers in chronic chlamydial infections than IgG are [59, 61]. IgA can also be measured from local secretions (e.g. excretions in chronic respiratory diseases), in which case they can be more illustrative, giving clues to what is happening in the areas in question (von Hertzen, to be published).

Micro-Immunofluorescence (Micro-IF)

Micro-IF has provided the first evidence of the possible association of *C. pneumoniae*, not only with acute [57], but also with chronic inflammatory processes [7, 26, 58]. If read with expertise and patience it can differentiate between the specific reactions and various interfering noises from cross-reacting antibodies to other chlamydial or bacterial species [23]. The necessity of an experienced reader is the weak point of the test. Moreover, the reading conditions must be strictly adjusted and patients must be tested with simultaneous titrations for locality, time, age, sex and social class-matched controls, both being read blindfolded by the same reader. In a subjective test like micro-IF no exact numerical values can be given: the result depends, besides on the reader, on the microscope and on the reagents used. Unfortunately, at the moment there is no standardised quality control system to check the performance of chlamydial micro-IF in different laboratories. Lacking that, the results published from various laboratories should be interpreted with some caution.

Unspecific Serological Tests. Unspecific test systems, like particle, LPS-EIA, and inclusion-based serological tests, being broad-reactive and sensitive to the common antigens presented in the course of chronic infections, are, paradoxically, perhaps more sensitive in monitoring chronic chlamydial infections. However, various different chronic chlamydial infections, due to as yet undiscovered species, can obscure the findings.

Immunoblotting. Immunoblotting offers the possibility of measuring specific responses to various chlamydial antigens [13, 20, 34]. The precise degree of specificity of the reactions is controversial since chlamydial proteins possess common epitopes which are exposed and reactive after PAGE-electrophoresis. However, these studies should be continued further in order to find the specific reactive proteins in chronic chlamydial infections [10,11,47, 51, 52]. These proteins or the synthetic peptides derived from them, could then be used in EIA to detect possible patients with persistent infection.

Immune Complexes

Immune complexes are produced in the battle against infecting organisms and generally consist of degradation products of the microbe and the respective antibodies bound to them. After healing, these complexes are gradually removed from circulation. Their longstanding presence is a sign of a continuous production of new complexes inside the body, i.e. constant production of microbial antigens and thus a persistent infection. This kind of complexes are typical of chronic infections and well documented in many viral and bacterial chronic diseases. Two kinds of immune complexes have been reported in suspected chronic chlamydial infections: those containing chlamydial LPS and respective antibodies [42], the majority being naturally of the IgM type, and those containing antibodies against chlamydial proteins [43]. LPS immune complexes tell nothing about the site of the chronic infection, since the LPS are more mobile within the body and can pass through cell layers into circulation. No corresponding transport mechanism is known for bacterial proteins.

The presence of immune complexes of bacterial proteins and respective antibodies in the bloodstream suggests the actual presence of the agent in intimate association with the blood circulation. In the case of *Chlamydia*, the agent could be present within live circulating blood cells, in live endothelium [36a], or in the areas where damaged endothelium allows the release of chlamydial proteins, produced during a chronic infection, directly into the bloodstream. Immune complexes containing chlamydial proteins are not easy to measure. The LPS-EIAs are tricky to handle [42] and precipitation of complexed antibodies is easily contaminated with co-precipitating antibodies simulating true immune complexes.

Moreover, the presence of specific immune complexes does not tell the exact location of the chronic process, i.e. whether it is situated in the lungs or in the venous or arterial side of the circulation. However, a simplified test for specific immune complexes could perhaps tell which individuals are suspected of harbouring *Chlamydia* in their lungs or blood vessels. The test could then be carried out repeatedly to document whether it is a slow and spontaneously resolving process, or whether it progresses with continuous worsening.

Antigen Detection

Antigen detection has been shown to be more effective than isolation in chronic *C. trachomatis* infections [64]. In chronic *C. pneumoniae* infections, the major obstacle is that of obtaining representative samples from the deep-sited areas of proposed lesions. However, evidence of chronic *C. pneumoniae* infection with documented immunohistochemical methods has already been published [39, 40, 65]. Antigen detection from easily obtained immune complexes found in circulation does not appear to be as sensitive as antibody detection, but so far it has not been studied sufficiently.

Nucleic Acid Detection

The promise for the future of exact diagnosis of chronic *C. pneumoniae* infections seems to lie in nucleic acid detection methods. The problems that still await a solution are: 1) how to obtain a proper sample; 2) how to process it in order to extract reactive nucleic acids in appropriate conditions; 3) how to neutralise interfering components in a biological sample; and 4) how to exclude the contamination of the extremely sensitive test system. *In situ* hybridization can, moreover, tell us about the exact location of a chronic *C. pneumoniae* infection. The problems are, hopefully, solvable, and nucleic acid detection methods applied to chronic infections may, in future, shed light on the problems associated with chronic chlamydial infections in a broader sense [14, 39].

Diseases Associated with a Chronic *C. pneumoniae* Infection

Chronic Bronchitis

Chronic bronchitis is the disease which immediately comes to mind when looking for possible chronic *C. pneumoniae* infections. To prove this on a basis of comparative antibody studies alone is difficult since patients are usually elderly men with a smoking habit, both of which factors tend to give high antibody prevalence [27,36,55]. In the first published study on the matter, no significant difference in IgG antibodies against *C. pneumoniae* was found between patients and age-matched controls [1]. However, Blasi et al. [6,7] found serological evidence that *C. pneumoniae* was participating in the process of chronic bronchitis exacerbations. Roos et al. [55] found no differences in serum IgG antibodies between patients and controls, but the difference in serum IgA prevalences was significant. Moreover, local sputum IgA antibodies against *C. pneumoniae*, absent in the majority of pneumonia patients sputa, were a common finding in the sputa of chronic bronchitis patients, along with local antibodies against *H. influenzae* and *B. catarrhalis* (von Hertzen, to be published). *C. pneumoniae* can therefore be added to the above mentioned bacteria which have invariably been associated with the pathogenesis of chronic bronchitis.

Asthma

It has been known for years that tetracyclines and macrolides have a therapeutic effect in some asthma cases, although this was explained by their general effect on leucocytes [46]. During later follow up studies on infants with *C. trachomatis* pneumonitis, asthma was found to be present in a third of former patients [74]. *C. pneumoniae* was associated with asthma by Hahn et al. [1, 8, 26, 30], who found the prevalence of adult onset asthma to be sevenfold more common after lower respiratory tract infection caused by *C. pneumoniae* than when compared to other causes. Prolonged macrolide treatment was effective in most cases where treatment had been started early in the disease [29]. Childhood asthma has also been associated with *C. pneumoniae*, and again macrolide treatment was found to be effective [18]. A persistent *C. pneumoniae* infection may participate in the asthmatic inflammation of the lungs and act as a co-factor in asthmatic episodes. This possibility should be thouroughly studied since the prevalence of asthma is globally increasing, even in areas without air pollution. It is tempting to speculate that the situation of a cortisone treatment in asthma would then be analogous to the use of gastric proton pump inhibitors in duodenal ulcer: symptoms are prevented, but a *Helicobacter pylori* infection persists.

Sarcoidosis

Sarcoidosis is a chronic inflammatory process of unknown origin with giant cell and granuloma formation, eventually resulting in scarring, and leading to tissue destruction. Refvem et al. [54] first noticed elevated chlamydial CF antibodies in association with sarcoidosis. Persistently elevated *C. pneumoniae* antibody titers were noted in sarcoidosis [24] and these were later studied in detail [52]. Sarcoidosis has been associated with acute episodes of *C. pneumoniae* infection [12, 24] as with other chlamydial lower respiratory tract infections [16, 32]. *C. pneumoniae* is able to survive and replicate within alveolar macrophages [3], and macrophage products such as ACE (angiotensin converting enzyme) and LZM (lysozyme), used to monitor the activity of sarcoidosis, correlated positively with *C. pneumoniae* micro-IF titers [24]. Theoretically, *C. pneumoniae* might thus initiate a process involved in the pathogenesis of sarcoidosis. Granuloma formation would then be analogous to that found in lymphogranuloma venereum caused by *C. trachomatis* LGV biovars.

However, in sarcoidosis many antibody titers are elevated and demonstration of the agent in affected tissue is needed before the association between sarcoidosis and *C. pneumoniae* can be confirmed.

Other Respiratory Tract Diseases

The extent of *C. pneumoniae* involvement in chronic conditions of the upper respiratory tract has not been fully addressed. Japanese workers have recently reported isolations of the agent both from acute and from chronic secretory otitis media [50]. Studies on chronic sinusitis have not been published so far. There is only one mention, in a limited study, of chronic interstitial pneumonitis [2] but no definite results were presented.

Immunological Complications

Erythema Nodosum

Starting from the first published report of a *C. pneumoniae* epidemic, the occurence of erythema nodosum, an immunological vasculitis, was noted [38, 57]. Erythema nodosum has been associated with respiratory chlamydial infections since 1965 [60], and some reports of this disease in connection with a *C. pneumoniae* infection have already appeared [19, 67]. Since *C. pneumoniae* is a common cause of disease, a search for a *C. pneumoniae* infection is recommended in every erythema nodosum case.

Reactive Arthritis

Chlamydia are common triggers of reactive arthritis [41]. The role played by *C. pneumoniae* as a cause of reactive arthritis has not yet been discovered for two main reasons: first, the complete recognition of the agent was reached quite recently; secondly, *C. trachomatis* is a cause of urethritis and conjunctivis besides reactive arthritis, and rheumatologists usually look for a sexually transmitted *Chlamydia* in these forms of arthritis. However, recent reports seem to indicate that *C. pneumoniae* is a common agent in reactive arthritis, which tends to appear after a respiratory tract infection [9, 22, 56]. Prolonged antibiotic treatment is effective against *C. trachomatis* induced reactive arthritis [41] and further studies are indicated in *C. pneumoniae* associated reactive arthritis.

Chronic Fatigue Syndrome

Prolonged convalescence is a typical sequelae in chlamydial pneumonias. In the Helsinki Heart Study an inverse correlation was noted between *C. pneumoniae* antibodies (and/or immune complexes) and sparetime physical activity (Leinonen et al., to be published). In one study on *C. pneumoniae* no correlation with IgG antibodies was found in chronic fatigue patients [37].

Chronic Cardiovascular Diseases

Cardiomyopathy

Sutton et al. [68] described a three year epidemic of cardiomyopathy in Illinois, with an exceptional feature of elevated chlamydial CF antibodies. The epidemic did not fit in with psittacosis/ornithosis but resembled a *C. pneumoniae* epidemic in its course. It is as yet unclear whether a cardiotropic strain [4] of *C. pneumoniae* or an unknown human chlamydial strain was responsible for the event. *C. pneumoniae* has been associated with subacute myocarditis found in Swedish elite orienteers [76].

Arteriosclerosis

Chlamydia has been associated with arteriosclerosis for about 50 years [25]. In the 1930s psittacosis was noted for embolic complications and cardiac inflammations and chlamydiae are now well established as a cause of several forms of cardites [49]. In the 1940s South American researchers found that in arteriosclerosis the intradermal Frei test, measuring hypersensitivity to all chlamydial species, was often positive without a history of LGV [17, 44, 53].

The association was rediscovered in Finland nearly 50 years later, when it was found that during acute myocardial infarction (AMI) a seroconversion against an epitope of chlamydial LPS could be demonstrated [58]. Further studies found that patients with AMI as well as those with coronary heart disease (CCHD) had stable elevated IgG and IgA titres against *C. pneumoniae* with the micro-immunofluorescence test. This led to the suggestion that the majority of AMI cases in Finland were associated with an exacerbation of chronic *C. pneumoniae* infection, which was also connected with CCHD. Seroconversions might be a sign of a sudden imbalance in relative amounts of chlamydial LPS and antibodies against this antigen [58]. The association between elevated antibody titres against *C. pneumoniae* and arteriosclerosis has been verified in three American studies [45,70,71], in a Swedish study [31], and in a study where smoking was a confounding factor [27, 28].

Immune complexes were found in about 60 % of the patients with AMI, and during convalescence from the disease the immune complex pattern shifted from antigen excess to antibody excess, showing a behaviour similar to the seroconversion noted earlier for LPS-EIA [42]. To verify the hypothesis of a chronic chlamydial infection caused by *C. pneumoniae*, precipitated immune complexes were analysed. Specific antibodies against *C. pneumoniae* proteins but not other *chlamydia* species were found in the precipitates [43]. The presence of immune complexes containing bacterial proteins is strong evidence in favour of the hypothesis that a chronic *C. pneumoniae* infection is situated in intimate association with the lumen of blood vessels and is, thus, continuously able to shed components directly into the blood circulation.

A study of the sera from a large prospective study on AMI, the Helsinki Heart Study (HHS), carried out on hypercholesteraemic men excluded the possibility that CCHD makes a person more vulnerable to *C. pneumoniae* infection, or that AMI only activates a latent *C. pneumoniae* infection. Over 4000 men were divided into cholesterol-lowering drug (gemfibrozil) or placebo treatment groups and followed for 5 years for the cardiac end-point [21]. Elevated IgG and/or IgA antibody titres and/or presence of immune complexes were associated with the fulfillment of the cardiac end-point up to 3-6 months earlier, constituting a 2.6-fold risk factor (CI 1.3 to 5.2), independent from classical risk factors.Those who had both steady high titres at the beginning and at the end of the study, suggesting a continuous chronic infection, were at higher risk for an AMI attack [59].

The independent new risk factor had joint effects with age and smoking (Leinonen et al., to be published). Smoking can lower defence mechanisms and thus aggravate a chronic chlamydial infection [27, 28, 36]. However, an unexpected finding was that the hypercholesteraemic men on the cholesterol lowering drug and with markers for simultaneous chronic *C. pneumoniae* infection were in greater danger. In this group, three to six months before the cardiac end-point, there was a sevenfold risk (Leinonen et al., to be published). In the gemfibrozil group the underlying background noise due to lipid anormalities (very prominent in this subgroup, recruited from hypercholesteraemic men), was perhaps diminished by the treatment and the underlying chronic *C. pneumoniae* infection was revealed in all its significance as a risk factor.

Other mechanisms may also be involved. Gram-negative septic infections have been known for a long time as being capable of inducing elevated triglyceridaemia and low high-density lipoprotein (HDL) values. These lipid alterations are particularly striking in *C. pneumoniae* pneumonia, despite the low mortality and benign outcome of the disease (Kauppinen et al., to be published). The above lipid pattern is a typical risk factor for CHD.

The Hsp 60 heat shock protein is an important factor in chronic chlamydial infections, causing cross-reactive autoimmunity antibodies [47]. These antibodies are found in patients with advanced carotid atheromatous lesions [77], and could well have developed against the *C. pneumoniae* Hsp 60 protein [5].

Demonstration of *C. pneumoniae* in Atherosclerotic Lesions

Shor et al. [65] realised that the curious double-layered vescicles with dense inner core, seen in atherosclerotic lesions with an electron microscope might be *C. pneumoniae* elementary bodies [15]. Their presence and identity were further verified by immunohistochemistry and nucleic acid detection by the Seattle group [39], which documented their presence in atheromatous lesions in the USA too [40]. Moreover, *C. pneumoniae* was not found in healthy areas of arterial wall. Whether or not the elementary bodies detected are inactive and are simply deposited within the lesions is as yet unknown. Since arteriosclerosis is a chronic inflammatory process [35], a chronic chlamydial infection participating in the process is strongly suggested.

C. pneumoniae and the Epidemiology of AMI

Chlamydia in vertebrates thrive in the intestinal tract [66], and the main route of non-venereal transmission of *C. psittaci* is faecal. Even *C. trachomatis* causes an intestinal infection in young infants, the agent being found in rectal specimens [63]. Bearing this in mind, it is interesting to note that in infection experiments carried out on monkeys *C. pneumoniae* was found in rectal swabs for prolonged periods [33]. There is a possibility that a faecal-oral cycle could be an alternative route to aerosol transmission via the respiratory tract for *C. pneumoniae*, particularly in crowded conditions with poor hygiene. The creation of a chronic *C. pneumoniae* focus on the mucous membranes, commonly colonized by Gram-negative organisms, in early childhood could possibly create a sort of respiratory tract mucosal immunity. The formation of a focus on the lung alveolus, so intimately connected with the circulation, would then be prevented. One can even speculate that improved hygiene in industrialized countries at the turn of the century has created another "polio story", now concerning an agent adapting to respiratory tract transmission, causing pneumonia in adults, and then leading to chronic infections with cardiovascular dissemination. Moreover, there can be profound differences in the immune response of children to a primary infection with *C. pneumoniae* when compared to primary infection in immunologically fully mature adults. Could it be that nowadays *C. pneumoniae* is perhaps adapting itself as a childhood respiratory disease? As a consequence, in crowded conditions with good hygienic standards, the incidence of asthma would perhaps increase, and coronary heart disease would be higher in developed countries in the areas where population is scarce enough to lead to a primary *C. pneumoniae* infection in adulthood.

Future Perspectives

Two of the chronic disease entities listed above, namely cardiovascular diseases and chronic obstructive pulmonary diseases, along with pneumonia, are amongst the six big killers of the world (WHO 1991). If the role of *C. pneumoniae* in these conditions can be proven, a revolution in their therapy may then follow. We have, at present, numerous chemotherapeutic drugs effective against the agent. (Incidentally, when these drugs appeared on the market CHD figures started to decrease). Intervention studies are therefore indicated for the close future; if their outcome is favourable, certain problems will still have to be solved. For example, we do not know whether early treatment with an effective drug will prevent a chronic infection from developing, and if so at what degree of mildness would the treatment then be indicated. If a chronic condition develops, we have no tool to diagnose those patients, within the vast majority with only a serological scar from a former

C. pneumoniae infection, who are at a risk of progressing towards irreparable damages. And if a good marker were found, we do not know what the therapeutic agent and the length of the treatment should be. There are currently no narrow-spectrum chlamydiocidic or even chlamydiostatic chemotherapeutic agents, and massive prolonged administration of current broad-spectrum *Chlamydia* antibiotics could have disastrous consequences on chemotherapy in a broader sense, with sudden upsurgence of bacterial resistance. Further studies are, therefore, urgently needed. An effective vaccine would be an ideal answer to the problem, but so far a vaccine does not even exist for *C. trachomatis*, despite 30 years' efforts. However, the knowledge collected in these studies can hopefully also be applied for the development of a *C. pneumoniae* vaccine.

References

1. Allegra L, Blasi F, Centanni S, Cosentini R, Denti F, Raccanelli R, Tarsia P, Valenti V (1994) Acute exacerbations of asthma in adults: role of *Chlamydia pneumoniae* infection. Eur Respir J 7:2165-2168
2. Beaty CD, Grayston JT, Wang SP, Kuo CC, Reto CS, Martin TR (1991) *Chlamydia pneumoniae*, strain TWAR, infection in patients with chronic obstructive pulmonary disease. Am Rev Respir Dis 144:1408-1410
3. Black CM, Perez R (1990) *Chlamydia pneumoniae* multiplies within human alveolar macrophages. In: Abstract of 90th Annual Meeting of A.S.M., Washington DC, American Society for Microbiology, 80
4. Black CM, Johnson JE, Farshy CE, Brown TM, Berdal BP (1991) Antigenic variation among strains of *Chlamydia pneumoniae*. J Clin Microbiol 29:1312-1316
5. Blanchard T, Bailey R, Holland M, Mabey D (1993) *Chlamydia pneumoniae* and atherosclerosis. Lancet 341:825 (letter)
6. Blasi F, Legnani D, Negretto GG, Caratozzolo O, Magliano E, Chiodo F, Pozzoli R, Fasoli A (1992) Incidence and prevalence of *Chlamydia pneumoniae* infection in COAD patients. J Infection 25 [Suppl 1]:125-126
7. Blasi F, Legnani D, Lombardo VM, Negretto GG, Magliano E, Pozzoli R, Chiodo F, Fasoli A , Allegra L (1993) *Chlamydia pneumoniae* infection in acute exacerbations of COPD. Eur Respir J 6:19-22
8. Bone RC (1991) *Chlamydia pneumoniae* and asthma. A potentially important relationship. JAMA 266:265 (editorial)
9. Braun J, Laitko S, Treharne J, Eggens U, Wu P, Distler A. Sieper J (1994) *Chlamydia pneumoniae*- a new causative agent of reactive arthritis and undifferenziated oligoarthritis. Ann Rheumat Dis 53:100-105
10. Brunham RC, Binns B, McDowell J, Paraskeva M (1986) *Chlamydia trachomatis* infection in women with ectopic pregnancy. Obstet Gynecol 67:722-726
11. Brunham RC, Peeling R, Maclean I, Kosseim ML, Paraskeva M (1992) *Chlamydia trachomatis* associated ectopic pregnancy: serologic and histologic correlates. J Infect Dis 165:1076-1081
12. Campbell JF, Barnes RC, Kozarsky PE, Spika JS (1991) Culture-confirmed pneumonia due to *Chlamydia pneumoniae*. J Infect Dis 164:411-413
13. Campbell LA, Kuo CC, Wang SP, Grayston JT (1990) Serological response to *Chlamydia pneumoniae* infection. J Clin Microbiol 28:1261-1264

14. Campbell LA, Patton DL, Moore DE, Cappuccio AL, Mueller BA, Wang SP (1993) Detection of *Chlamydia trachomatis* DNA in women with tubal infertility. Fertil Steril 59:45-50

15. Chi EY, Kuo CC, Graystone JT (1987) Unique ultrastructure in the elementary bodiey of *Chlamydia sp.* strain TWAR. J Bacteriol 169:3757-3763

16. Crosse BA, Gomes P, Muers MM (1991) Ovine psittacosis and sarcoidosis in a pregnant woman. Thorax 46:604-606

17. Coutts WE, Davila M (1945) Lymphogranuloma venereum as a possible cause of arteriosclerosis and other arterial condition. J Trop Med Hyg 48:46-51

18. Emre U, Roblin P, Gellin M, Dumornay W, Rao M, Hammerschlag M, Shacter J (1994) The association of *C. pneumoniae* infection and reactive airway disease in children. Arch Pediatr Adolesc Med 148:727-732

19. Erntell M, Ljunggren K, Gadd T, Persson K (1989) Erythema nodosum- a manifestation of *Chlamydia pneumoniae* (strain TWAR) infection. Scand J Infect Dis 21:693-696

20. Freidank HM, Herr AS, Jacobs E (1993) Identification of *C. pneumoniae*-specific protein antigens in immunoblots. Eur J Clin Microbiol Infect Dis 12:947-951

21. Frick MH, Elo O, Haapa K, Heinonen OP, Heinsalmi P, Helo P, Hutten JK, Kaitaniemi P et al (1987) Helsinki Heart Study: Primary-prevention trial with genfibrozil in middle aged men with dyslipidemia. Safety of treatment, changes in risk factors, and incidence of coronary heart disease. N Engl J Med 317:1237-1245

22. Gran JT, Hjetland R, Andreassen AH (1993) Pneumonia, myocarditis and reactive arthritis due to *Chlamydia pneumoniae*. Scand J Rheumatol 22:43-44

23. Grayston JT, Golubjatnikov R, Hagiwara T, Hahn DL, Leinonen M, Persson K, Saikku P, Treharne J, Wang SP (1993) Serologic tests for *Chlamydia pneumonaie*. Pediatr Infect Dis 11:790-791

24. Grönhagen-Riska C, Saikku P, Riska H, Fröseth B, Grayston JT (1988) Antibodies to TWAR - a novel Type of *Chlamydia* - in sarcoidosis. In: Sarcoidosis and other granulomatous disorders Grassi C et al (eds), Elsevier Scientific Publ, Amsterdam, pp 297-301

25. Haagen E (1964) Miyagawallen. In: Viruskrankheiten des Menschen, Band I, Dietrich Steikopff Verlag, Darmstadt, pp 807-1052

26. Hahn DL, Dodge RW, Golubjatnikov R (1991) Association of *Chlamydia pneumoniae* (strain TWAR) infection with wheezing, asthmatic bronchitis, and adult-onset asthma. JAMA 266:225-230

27. Hahn DL, Golubjatnikov R (1992) Smoking is a potential confounder of the *Chlamydia pneumoniae*-coronary heart disease association. Arterioscler Thrombosis 12:945-947

28. Hahn DL, Sikku P, Leinonen M, Tenkanen L (1992) *Chlamydia*, smoking, and heart disease. Ann Int Med 117:171

29. Hahn DL (1993) Clinical experience with anti-chlamydial therapy for adult onset of asthma. Am Rev Respir Dis 147:A297

30. Hahn DL, Golubjatnikov R (1994) Adult onset asthma and atypical infection: a case series. J Family Pract 38:1-7

31. Haidl S, Juul-Müller, Israelsson B, Persson K (1992) Ischemic heart disease and antibodies to *Chlamydia pneumoniae* (TWAR). Proc European Soc for Chlamydia Res 2:174

32. Harris AA, Pottage JC Jr, Kessler HA, Zeihen M, Levin S (1984) *Psittacosis bacteriemia* in a patient with sarcoidosis. Ann Intern Med 101:502-503

33. Holland SM, Taylor HR, Gaydoa CA, Kappus EW, Quinn TC (1990) Experimental infection with *Chlamydia pneumoniae* in non-human primates. Infect Immun 58:593-597

34. Iijima Y, Miyashita N, Kishimoto T, Kanamoto Y, Soejima R, Matsumoto A (1994) Characterization of *Chlamydia pneumoniae* species specific proteins immunodominant in humans. J Clin Microbiol 32:583-588

35. Jang IK, Lassila R, Fuster V (1993) Atherogenesis and inflammation. Eur Heart J 14 [Suppl K]:2-6

36. Karvonen M, Tuomilehto J, Pitkäniemi J, Naukkarinen A, Saikku P (1994) Importance of smoking for *Chlamydia pneumoniae* infection. Int J Epidemiol 23:1315-1321

36a. Kaukoranta-Tolvanen SS, Laitinen K, Saikku P, Leinonen M (1994) *Chlamydia pneumoniae* multiplies in endothelial cells in vitro. Microbiol Pathogen 16:313-319

37. Komaroff AL, Wang SP, Lee J, Grayston JT (1992) No association of chronic *Chlamydia pneumoniae* infection with chronic fatigue syndrome. J Infect Dis 165:182

38. Kousa M, Saikku P, Kanerva L (1980) Erythema nodosum in chlamydial infections. Acta Dermatovener, Stockolm, 60:319-322

39. Kuo CC, Shor A, Campbell LA, Fukushi H, Patton DL, Grayston JT (1993) Demonstration of *Chlamydia pneumoniae* in atherosclerotic lesions of coronary arteries. J Infect Dis 167:845-849

40. Kuo CC, Gown AM, Benditt EP, Grayston JT (1993) Detection of *Chlamydia pneumoniae* in aortic lesions of atherosclerosis by immunocytochemical stain. Arterioscler Thromb 13:1501-1504

41. Lauhio A, Leirisalo-Repo M, Lähdevirta J, Saikku P, Repo H (1991) Double-blind, placebo-controlled study of three month lymecycline course in reactive arthritis with special reference to *Chlamydia arthritis*. Arthritis Rheumatism 34:6-14

42. Leinonen M, Linnanmäki E, Mattila K, Nieminen MS, Leirisalo-Repo M, Valtonen V, Saikku P (1990) Circulating immune complexes containing chlamydial lypopolisaccharide in acute myocardial infarction. Microbial Pathogenesis 9:67-73

43. Linnanmärki E, Leinonen M, Ekman MR, Mattila K, Nieminen MS, Valtonen V, Saikkui P (1993) *Chlamydia pneumoniae* specific circulating immune complexes in chronic heart disease Circulation 87:1130-1134

44. May J (1943) La intradermoreaccion de Frei en las arteropatias. Rev Argentina Dermatosifil 27:581-582

45. Melnick SL, Shahar E, Folsom AR, Grayston JT, Sorlie PD, Wang SP, Szklo M (1993) Past infection by *C. pneumoniae* strain TWAR and asymptomatic carotid atherosclerosis. Am J Med 95:499-504

46. Miyataka H, Taki F, Taniguchi H, Suzuki R, Takagi K, Satake T (1991) Erythromycin reduces the severity of bronchial hyperresponsiveness in asthma. Chest 99:670-673

47. Morrison RP, Lyng K, Caldwell HD (1989) Chlamydial pathogenesis. Ocular hypersensitivity elicited by a genus specific 57 kDa protein. J Exp Med 169:663-675

48. Mårdh PA, Paavonen J, Puolakkainen M (1989) *Chlamydia*. Plenum Medical Book Co., New York and London, p 370

49. Odeh M, Oliven A (1992) Chlamydial infections of the heart. Eur J Clin Microbiol Infect Dis 11:885-893

50. Ogawa H, Hashiguchi K, Kazuyama Y (1992) Recovery of *C. pneumoniae* in six patients with otitis media with effusion. J Laryngol Otology 106:490-492

51. Puolakkainen M, Kuo CC, Shor A, Wang SP, Grayston JT, Campbell LA (1993) Serological response to *Chlamydia pneumoniae* in adults with coronary arterial fatty streaks and fibrolipid plaques. J Clin Microbiol 31:2212-2214

52. Puolakkainen M, Campbell LA, Kuo CC, Leinonen M, Grönhagen-Riska C, Saikku P (1993) Serological response to *C. pneumoniae* in patients with sarcoidosis. Abstr 93rd AMS Gen Meet, Washington DC

53. Quiroga, Ambrosetti FE (1943) La reaccion de Frei en las endoarterites obliterantes. Rev Argentina Dermatosifil 27:624-625

54. Refvem O, Bjornstad RT, Loe K (1976) The ornithosis complement fixation test in sar-

coidosis. Ann NY Acad Sci 278:225-228

55. Roos L, Leinonen M, Isoaho R, Koskinen R, Saikku P (1994) Serological evidence of persistent *Chlamydia pneumoniae* infection associated with chronic bronchitis. (submitted)

56. Saario R, Toivanen A (1973) *Chlamydia pneumoniae* as a cause of reactive arthritis. Clin Rheumatol 11:161

57. Saikku P, Wang SP, Kleemola M, Brander E, Rusanen E, Grayston JT (1985) An epidemic of mild pneumonia due to an unusual strain of *Chlamydia psittaci*. J Infect Dis 151:832-839

58. Saikku P, Mattila K, Nieminen MS, Hutten JK, Leinonen M, Ekman MR, Makela PH, Valtona V (1988) Serological evidence of an association of a novel *Chlamydia*, TWAR, with chronic heart disease and acute myocardial infarction Lancet ii:983-985

59. Saikku P, Leinonen M, Tenkanen L, Ekman MR, Linnanmärki E, Manninen V, Mänttäri M, Frick MM, Huttunen JK (1992) Chronic *Chlamydia pneumoniae* infection as a risk factor for coronary heart disease in the Helsinki Heart Study Ann Int Med 116:273-278

60. Sarner M, Wilson RJ (1965) Erythema nodosum and psittacosis: report of five cases. Brit Med J 2:1469-1470

61. Sarov I, Sarov B, Hanuka N, Glasner M, Kaneti J (1986) The significance of serum specific IgA antibodies in diagnosis of active *Chlamydia trachomatis* infections. In: Chlamydial Infections, Oriel D et al (eds), Cambridge University Press, Cambridge, pp 566-569

62. Schacter J, Smith DE, Dawson CR, Anderson WR, Deller JJ, Hoke AW, Smartt WH, Meyer KF (1969) Lymphogranuloma venereum. Comparison of Frei test, complement fixation test, and isolation of the agent. J Infect Dis 120:372-375

63. Schacter J, Grossman M, Holt J, Sweet R, Spector S (1979) Infection with *Chlamydia trachomatis*: involvement of multiple anatomic sites in neonates. J Infect Dis 139:232-234

64. Schacter J, Moncada J, Dawson CR, Sheppard J, Courtright P, Said ME, Zaki S, Hafez SF, Lorincz A (1988) Nonculture methods for diagnosing chlamydial infection in patients with trachoma: a clue to the pathogenesis of the disease? J Infect Dis 158:1347-1352

65. Shor A, Kuo CC, Patton DL (1992) Detection of *Chlamydia pneumoniae* in coronary arterial fatty streaks and atheromatous plaques. S Afr Med J 82:158-161

66. Storz J (1971) Intestinal chlamydial infections in ruminant. In: Chlamydia and Chlamydia induced Diseases. Charles Thomas, Springfield, IL, pp.146-154

67. Sundelöf B, Gnarpe H, Gnarpe J (1993) An unusual manifestation of *Chlamydia pneumoniae* infection: meningitis, hepatitis, iritis and atypical erythema nodosum. Scand J Infect Dis 25:259-261

68. Sutton GC, Demakis JA, Anderson A, Morrisey RA (1971) Serologic evidence of a sporadic outbreak in Illinois of infection by *Chlamydia* (psittacosis-LGV agent) in patients with primary myocardial disease and respiratory disease. Am Heart J 81:597-607

69. Syrjälä H, Saikku P, Leinonen M, Airaksinen J, Surcel HM *Chlamydia pneumoniae* specific cell-mediated immunity in coronary heart disease. (Submitted)

70. Thom DH, Wang SP, Grayston JT, Siscovick DS, Stewart DK, Konmal RA, Weiss NS (1991) *Chlamydia pneumoniae* strain TWAR antibody and angiographically demonstrated coronary artery disease. Arteriosclerosis Thromb 11:547-551

71. Thom DH, Grayston JT, Siscovick DS,Wang SP, Weiss NS, Daling JR (1992) Association of prior infection with *Chlamydia pneumoniae* and angiographically demonstrated coronary artery disease. JAMA 268:68-72

72. Wang SP, Grayston JT (1982) Microimmunofluorescence antibody responses in *Chlamydia trachomatis* infection, a review. In: Chlamydial infections. Märdh PA et al (eds), Elsevier Biomed Press, Amsterdam, pp 301-316

73. Wang SP, Grayston JT (1986) Microimmunofluorescence serological studies with the

TWAR organism. In: Chlamydial Infections, Oriel D et al (eds), Cambridge University Press, Cambridge, pp 329-332

74. Weiss SG, Newcomb RW, Beem MO (1986) Pulmonary assessment of children after chlamydial pneumonia of infancy. J Pediatr 108:659-664

75. Weiss S, Roblin P, Gaydos C, Schulhoff N, Shani J, Quinn T, Hammershlag M, Schacter J (1993) Failure to isolate *Chlamydia pneumoniae* from coronary atheroma in patients undergoing atherectomy. Abstr 33rd ICAAC, New Orleans, Oct 17-20 1993, No. 1596 p 411

76. Wesslen L, Paholson G, Friman G, Fohlman J, Lindquist O, Johansson C (1992) Myocarditis caused by *Chlamydia pneumoniae* (TWAR) and sudden unexpected death in a Swedish elite orienteer. Lancet 340:427-428

77. Xu Q, Willeit J, Marosi M, Kleindienst R, Oberhollenzer F, Kiechl S, Stulnig T, Luff G, Wick G (1993) Association of serum antibodies to heat-shock protein 65 with carotid atherosclerosis. Lancet 341:255-259

Chapter 9   Evidence for *Chlamydia pneumoniae* Infection in Asthma

DAVID L. HAHN

Introduction

According to the British Thoracic Society, "asthma is a common and chronic inflammatory condition of the airways whose cause is not completely understood" [1]. Two important clinical characteristics of asthma are: 1) *reversible airway obstruction*, usually manifested by complaints of episodic cough, wheeze, shortness of breath and/or chest tightness, and 2) *bronchial hyperreactivity to a variety of stimuli* including aeroallergens, irritants, cold air, exercize and respiratory infections which can exacerbate or trigger asthma symptoms in susceptible individuals [2]. Asthma is a common medical condition affecting approximately 5-10% of children and adults worldwide [3] and is an important cause of morbidity in all age groups and mortality especially in the elderly [4].

An important recent advance in the understanding of asthma pathophysiology is the recognition that asthma, even in its earliest stages, is associated with chronic inflammation of the airways [5]. Bronchial inflammation appears to be necessary but not sufficient to produce asthma symptoms, which seem to occur only in susceptible individuals, possibly related to genetic acquisition of bronchial hyperreactivity [6]. Thus, asthma may be succinctly characterized as a chronic inflammatory condition of unknown etiology [2].

Because its underlying causes are unknown, asthma must be regarded as a syndrome, not a disease. Although IgE-mediated childhood allergy to common aeroallergens (mites, molds, plants, animal dander, etc.) has become synonymous with asthma in the public consciousness, this type of *allergic* or *atopic* asthma represents only one of several recognized asthma syndromes [7]. A substantial amount of asthma first becomes apparent in adulthood [8], and adult-onset asthma is not uniformly associated with IgE-mediated positive skin test reactions to common aeroallergens [9]. A significant but incompletely quantified proportion of childhood asthma is also not strongly associated with atopy [7].

Burrows et al. [9] recently reported that skin test-negative adult-onset asthma is nevertheless associated with increased levels of serum IgE and blood eosinophils, leading these investigators and others [10, 11] to postulate the existence of a missing antigen (not included in the batteries of common aeroallergens used for skin testing), potentially responsible for producing increased serum IgE levels and eosinophilia in "nonatopic" (skin test negative) asthma patients. Evidence supports the concept that a final common pathophysiologic pathway for both atopic and non-atopic asthma syndromes involves eosinophilic inflammation in asthmatic airways [12]. This chapter reviews current evidence regarding whether and to what extent *Chlamydia pneumoniae* infection is responsible for producing this postulated *missing antigen*.

Historical Views of Asthma Etiology

Fifty years ago many clinicians believed that asthma was primarily infectious in nature, that allergy was of secondary importance [13-15] and that the primary consideration in management was the treatment of bronchitis accompanying asthma [15, 16]. However, relatively little scientific evidence has accumulated implicating infection as an underlying cause for asthma [17]. A role for viral infections as exacerbating (trigger) factors in asthma attacks is widely acknowledged, but current expert opinion does not recognize a role for bacterial infection as an underlying cause in the initiation or promotion of asthma [2]. If current evidence, reviewed here, associating *C. pneumoniae* infection with the initiation, exacerbation and promotion of asthma is confirmed, our view of infection as a cause for asthma may need to be revised yet again.

Serologic Evidence: Clinical

C. pneumoniae polyvalent (mixture of IgM, IgG, IgA) seroreactivity was first associated with wheezing, asthmatic bronchitis and adult-onset asthma in a study designed to assess the etiologic roles of *C. pneumoniae, C. trachomatis* and *Mycoplasma pneumoniae* in community-acquired acute lower respiratory illnesses [18]. In this study of 365 adults with acute respiratory illness, asthma symptoms were noted in 9 (47%) of 19 adult patients with acute *C. pneumoniae* infection (mostly reinfection) diagnosed by serologic methods. In addition to asthma symptoms described in patients with acute infection, both wheezing during acute illness and the diagnosis of asthmatic bronchitis within six months post-enrollment were strongly associated in a dose-dependent fashion with *C. pneumoniae* polyvalent titer magnitude in patients not meeting criteria for acute infection. Finally, some patients in this study developed chronic asthma for the first time following acute *C. pneumoniae* infection, and antibiotic treatment appeared to be effective in alleviating symptoms of asthma. There were no comparable associations of asthma with serologic evidence for *M. pneumoniae, C. trachomatis* or respiratory viral infections, although rhinovirus was not studied. The Authors concluded that some *C. pneumoniae* titers, although not diagnostic for acute infection, probably represented reinfection or ongoing chronic infection. They argued further that it was biologically plausible that repeated or prolonged exposure to *C. pneumoniae* could cause the airway inflammation known to occur in asthma [18].

Table 1 presents additional serologic data derived from an expanded cohort of 450 primary care outpatients including those reviewed above [18]. Since the original published study [18] reported only on *C. pneumoniae* titers of 1:64 or greater, the

Table 1. Association of *Chlamydia pneumoniae* polyvalent antibody with (A) acute asthmatic bronchitis and (B) asthma

Titer category	(A) Acute asthmatic bronchitis			(B) Asthma		
		Crude OR	Adjusted OR (95% CI)*		Crude OR	Adjusted OR (95% CI)*
Seronegative	17/77 (22)**	1.0 (ref)	1.0 (ref)	2/87 (2)**	1.0 (ref)	1.0 (ref)
Nondiagnostic (1:16)	14/30 (47)	3.1	2.8 (1.0-7.7)	1/42 (2)	1.0	1.3 (.10-16.9)
Nondiagnostic (1:32)	17/37 (46)	3.0	3.1 (1.2-8.0)	4/53 (8)	3.5	6.9 (1.0-16.8)
Nondiagnostic (1:64)	10/21 (48)	3.2	3.4 (1.1-10.4)	3/24 (13)	6.1	9.0 (1.2-70.5)
Nondiagnostic (≥1:128)	16/22 (73)	9.4	10.5 (3.0-37.7)	4/14 (29)	17	21.1 (2.5-178)
Acute antibody	7/12 58	4.9	5.5 (4.3-23.9)	2/10 (20)	10.6	9.6 (.97-94.8)

* From logistic regression controlled for age, sex and smoking. For acute asthmatic bronchitis patients, controls were 118 concurrently enrolled patients with upper respiratory illnesses (pharyngitis, laryngitis and sinusitis). For asthma patients, controls were 214 concurrently enrolled patients with acute bronchitis who did not wheeze. Tests for trend in the odds ratios for both asthmatic bronchitis and asthma. $p<01$
** No. with asthmatic bronchitis or asthma/total patients (%)

analysis presented here addresses the question whether titers of 1:16 or 1:32 are also associated with clinical evidence for reactive airway diseases. As can be seen in Table 1, *C. pneumoniae* titers of 1:16 or greater were significantly associated with acute asthmatic bronchitis, whereas titers of 1:32 or greater were significantly associated with chronic asthma. In clinical practice, acute asthmatic bronchitis may be defined as symptoms and signs (usually wheezing) of acutely reversible airway obstruction (bronchospasm) in a patient with acute infectious bronchitis who does not have a previous history of chronic asthma [19]. A diagnosis of asthma implies longstanding symptoms of wheezing and shortness of breath which are not limited to episodes of acute respiratory infection.

Associations between *C. pneumoniae* antibody and asthma have been replicated and extended to include pulmonary function test-confirmed asthma and chronic obstructive pulmonary disease (COPD) in patient groups from the United States [20], Great Britain [21], Finland [22] and Italy [23]. Acute *C. pneumoniae* antibody has also been reported in acute exacerbations of asthma in adults who had *C. pneumoniae* identified in the oropharynx by means of a direct fluorescent antibody (DFA) test [23].

Preliminary data suggest that certain clinical characteristics may identify asthma patients likely to be seroreactive to *C. pneumoniae*. *C. pneumoniae* antibody-asthma associations have been described in patients without a personal or family history of clinical allergy (allergic rhinitis or eczema) [18]. Skin test positivity is usually associated with childhood-onset asthma, whereas *C. pneumoniae* antibody is more likely to be associated with skin test negative adult-onset asthma [24]. However, a role for *C. pneumoniae* infection in some cases of skin test-positive asthma is possible and needs further investigation [24].

An infectious presentation for asthma (asthma developing after bronchitis, pneumonia or an influenza-like illness) has been associated with *C. pneumoniae* polyvalent antibody in patients meeting American Thoracic Society (ATS) criteria for asthma [10]. This infectious presentation for asthma has also been associated with a serologic profile consisting of *C. pneumoniae*-specific IgG in a titer of 1:128 or greater in combination with an IgA titer of 1:16 or greater. Figure 1 presents data for 104 asthma patients (ATS criteria) in whom asthma clinical presentation (infectious/noninfectious) was classified before serologic results (IgG/IgA profile) were obtained. Infectious asthma was defined in patients reporting asthma beginning after an acute respiratory illness (bronchitis, pneumonia or an influenza-like illness) whereas noninfectious asthma was defined as atopic, occupational or exercize-induced asthma. The serologic profiles IgG<128/IgA<16 and IgG≥128/IgA≥16 predominated over the other two possible combinations in a non-random fashion ($p < 10^{-10}$) for this group of asthma patients. Most patients classified with noninfectious asthma

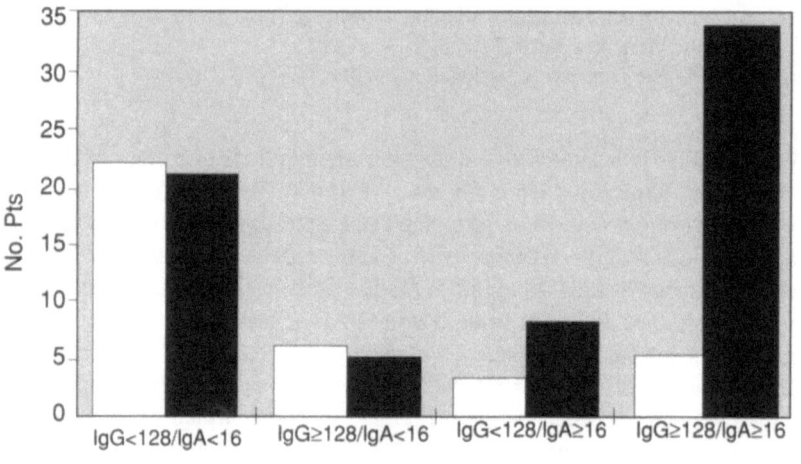

Chlamydia pneumoniae and infectious asthma

Fig. 1. Association of *Chlamydia pneumoniae* IgG /IgA serologic profiles with different clinical presentations for chronic asthma. Serologic profiles consisted of the four possible combinations of IgG less than 1:128 or IgG equal to or greater than 1:128 in combination with IgA less than 1:16 or equal to or greater than 1:16. Asthma (ATS criteria) diagnosed following acute respiratory illness (bronchitis, pneumonia or an influenza-like illness) was defined as infectious (black bars). Atopic, occupational and exercize-induced asthma are termed noninfectious (open bars). The *C. pneumoniae* serologic profile IgG≥128/IgA≥16 was significantly associated with infectious asthma ($p < 0.05$)

had the negative serologic category (IgG<128/IgA<16). Approximately one-third of patients classified with infectious asthma also had the serologic profile IgG<128/IgA<16. A substantial proportion of the remaining two-thirds of infectious asthma patients had the serologic profile IgG≥128/IgA≥16. The positive predictive value of the serologic profile IgG≥128/IgA≥16 for infectious asthma in this asthma patient group was 87%. High titer *C. pneumoniae* IgG and/or IgA seroreactivity has been associated with chronic *C. pneumoniae* infection in coronary artery disease [25]. The serologic profile IgG≥128/IgA≥16 has also been described by Falck et al. [26] in a case of adult bronchitis associated with persistent bronchial obstruction treated with inhaled steroids. Further studies will be required to determine whether the serologic profile IgG≥128/IgA≥16 predicts chronic chlamydial infection in asthma.

Thus, the proposed clinical profile for the asthma patient most likely to have serologic evidence for possible chronic chlamydial infection is the clinically nonallergic, skin test negative patient giving a history of adult-onset asthma beginning after respiratory illness. Other clinical presentations which may be associated with *C. pneumoniae* infection include adult patients with some accompanying clinical allergy and skin test positivity, as well as a less well-defined subgroup of children with asthma. Cough variant asthma as a presentation for *C. pneumoniae* infection has also been reported [27]. Further studies are required to confirm and refine these proposed clinical correlates of chlamydial asthma.

Seroepidemiologic Evidence

C. pneumoniae infection has been suggested as a possible explanation for increases in asthma noted in recent decades [28]. There are no published population-based epidemiologic studies to have addressed this possibility directly. However, *C. pneumoniae* and asthma prevalence data from the same geographic areas and similar time periods are available. Cross-sectional data show that the age-specific *C. pneumoniae* seroprevalence pattern [29] resembles the age-specific prevalence pattern of symptomatic adult asthma [30] documented for Denmark. Superimposition of these patterns [29, 30] reveals that the slope of the *C. pneumoniae* age-specific seroprevalence curve begins to increase approximately 10 years before a comparable rise in prevalence of symptomatic adult asthma is noted. A 5 to 10 year time interval has also been described for the development of secondary cases of asthma in other epidemiologic studies suggesting the involvement of a transmissable agent [31, 32].

Population-based longitudinal data from Finland indicate that an increasing *C. pneumoniae* seroprevalence rate [33] is associated with increases in asthma, particularly in middle-aged women and elderly men but also to some extent in children [34]. Ecologic data from Great Britain also show increasing *C. pneumoniae* seroprevalence rates in adults [35] as adult acute bronchitis and asthma increase, also in middle-aged females and elderly males [36]. Regarding the proportion of adult-onset asthma potentially attributable to *C. pneumoniae* infection, 100% of adult-onset asthmatics reported in a clinical seroepidemiologic study were *C. pneumoniae* seroreactive, compared to 53% seroreactivity in controls with non-wheezing respiratory illnesses [20].

Summary of the Serologic Evidence

Serologic evidence for *C. pneumoniae* infection has been found in: 1) acute asthmatic bronchitis in patients without chronic asthma [18, 20] 2) chronic asthma in younger adults without fixed obstruction [10, 20] and 3) chronic asthma in older adults with coexisting fixed obstruction [10, 20]. It is unknown whether previously described differences in epidemiology for asthma beginning before and after the age of 40 years [37, 38] represent different underlying etiologies for different diseases, or different clinical presentations for the same underlying disease etiology. If *C. pneumoniae* is proven to be a causal factor in the three clinical presentations for which serologic associations have been described, it may be surmised that chlamydial infection can produce different asthma clinical presentations at different ages.

Organism Identification in Asthma

An obvious limitation of serologic associations is the indirect nature of the evidence for infection. Ideally, serologic studies should be accompanied by isolation of the organism or direct identification by other means. In adults, *C. pneumoniae* has been cultured from cases of adult acute bronchitis with wheezing [39, 40] and from adults experiencing early acute phases of asthma [41] including steroid-treated asthma [42]. Inadvertant laboratory-acquired infection with *C. pneumoniae* has resulted in pneumonia followed by asthma (Saikku, personal communication).

C. pneumoniae has also been cultured from a proportion of prospectively enrolled inner city Brooklyn children with symptomatic asthma [43]. Another prospective, community-based cohort study of English children with asthma identified *C. pneumoniae* by polymerase chain reaction (PCR) testing in 46.9% of subjects (24% during exacerbations and 27.7% when asymptomatic) [44]. Since there was no association with acute exacerbations, this appears to be evidence for chronic infection in a surprisingly large subgroup of children with asthma. No comparable series of culture- or PCR-positive adult asthmatics have been published.

Treatment

It is important to know whether appropriate treatment of *C. pneumoniae* will hasten resolution of airway irritability associated with *C. pneumoniae* infection [45]. Antichlamydial antimicrobial therapy of asthma in groups of children [43] and adults [46] has resulted in improvement of asthma symptoms. Sometimes, asthma symptoms in treated patients have completely disappeared, and pulmonary function has normalized, resulting in prolonged remission of a condition believed to be incurable [47, 48]. These results have been demonstrated after open label, uncontrolled treatment of individual cases or of groups of patients with evidence of chlamydial infection. Larger, multicenter, randomized, controlled, double-blinded therapeutic trials of antichlamydial antimicrobial therapy of asthma will be required before final conclusions regarding the benefit of treatment can be made. Existing information is reviewed here.

During a prospective culture and serologic study of the association of *C. pneumoniae* infection and reactive airway disease, Emre et al [43] enrolled 118 inner city children between the ages of 5 and 16 years attending an emergency department because of exacerbations of asthma. Nine (7.6%) had positive nasopharyngeal cultures for *C. pneumoniae* but did not have antibody indicative of acute infection, 13 (11%) had acute antibody but were culture negative and 3 (2.5%) were positive by both culture and serology; one additional culture positive patient did not have a serologic specimen available. The 13 (11%) culture positive patients were treated with one or more courses of a macrolide and all eventually became culture negative. Nine (75%) had clinical and laboratory improvement in asthma after eradication of *C. pneumoniae*. Response to therapy was related to the severity of disease as all children with mild asthma improved whereas not all children with moderate or severe disease improved. The Authors hypothesized that chronic *C. pneumoniae* infection could produce chronic airway inflammation and bronchial hyperresponsiveness in susceptible individuals [43].

In adult cases, treatment of *C. pneumoniae* infection has produced improvement [18, 27] and complete remission [47, 48] of asthma. Two case reports of antichlamydial therapy in adult asthma are illustrative:

1. A skin test-negative 40 year old woman developed persistent asthma following an acute wheezing illness which was associated with serologic evidence for acute *C. pneumoniae* infection (IgM titer of 1:16). She had a complete two year remission of asthma symptoms following five weeks of doxycycline, 100 mg orally twice daily (three weeks were insufficient to eradicate symptoms). A relapse two years later was associated with serologic evidence of possible reinfection (polyvalent titer of 1:512 without an IgM response) and the patient had improvement after retreatment [47]. This case suggests that acute infection may persist in a chronic form to produce asthma symptoms, and that reinfection (or reactivation of latent infection) may cause reactivation of asthma.

2. Antichlamydial treatment resulted in improvement of cough variant asthma in a 39 year old man with elevated IgE and eosinophilia [27]. Pretreatment testing revealed a *C. pneumoniae* IgG titer of 1:1024, an IgA titer of 1:32 and an IgM titer of less than 1:8. This case suggests that cough variant asthma may be another clinical expression of *C. pneumoniae* infection, which may produce eosinophilia and elevated IgE in association with asthma.

Eosinophilia has also been reported in another patient with adult-onset asthma in whom *C. pneumoniae* was persistently isolated from the nasopharynx [48]. After antichlamydial antimicrobial therapy, *C. pneumoniae* was no longer cultivable from the nasopharynx, eosinophilia and asthma symptoms disappeared and pulmonary function was improved.

Prompt treatment of newly acquired chlamydial infections should prevent long-term inflammatory sequelae whereas treatment of late stage chlamydial disease would not be expected to offer as much benefit. A study of *C. pneumoniae* seroreactive adults with asthma is being conducted to determine whether improvement after antichlamydial treatment will be greater in recently symptomatic asthma patients compared to asthma patients with late-stage disease. Preliminary results in 24 patients showed that recently symptomatic asthma did respond more favorably than late asthma [46].

Currently, analysis of 48 treated patients confirms the preliminary findings (Hahn manuscript submitted). In this ongoing study, some treated patients with recently symptomatic asthma have had prolonged, complete remissions.

Treatment results have been much less dramatic in longstanding asthma with coexisting, fixed obstruction [19], suggesting that prompt recognition and early treatment may be necessary to benefit patients with chlamydial asthma.

The Chlamydia-Asthma Hypothesis

A variety of respiratory pathogens (particularly viruses and *Mycoplasma pneumoniae*) can cause exacerbations of asthma, but less is known about an infectious initiation or promotion of asthma [49]. During reinfection or chronic infection, *chlamydiae* produce T-cell mediated immunopathology and thus *C. pneumoniae* is hypothetically capable of long-term asthma promotion [18]. According to the chlamydia-asthma hypothesis, treatment of chronic *C. pneumoniae* infection should reduce or eliminate the burden of infection-associated antigens contributing to asthmatic inflammation and symptoms. The treatment results reviewed above support this hypothesis.

The limited data available are consistent with an estimate that *C. pneumoniae* infection could be etiologically associated with most adult-onset asthma, and with a lesser but still substantial proportion of childhood asthma. An important unproven hypothesis, worthy of serious consideration, is that a significant amount of asthma is related to chronic chlamydial infection.

Conclusions

Most basic research on asthma pathophysiology and treatment is currently focused "downstream" on the consequences of the inflammatory cascade in the asthmatic lung. Little research has been directed "upstream" towards primary causation.

Despite the introduction of more effective forms of anti-inflammatory therapy for asthma, recent unexplained worldwide increases in incidence, prevalence, morbidity and mortality for asthma have been documented [50]. There is also evidence that *C. pneumoniae* infection is increasing [33]. The evidence for chlamydial involvement in asthma reviewed here provides a plausible framework for future research into primary causation which might lead to new treatments or novel preventive stategies for this clinically important disease.

Acknowledgements

I wish to thank Roberta McDonald for performing serologic testing and for her helpful comments during preparation of this chapter. I also wish to express my gratitude to Lori Bakken, Mary Sanchez and Marty Skemp for their unflagging helpfulness in locating reference materials.

References

1. British Thoracic Society (1993) Guidelines on the management of asthma. Thorax 48 [Suppl]:1-24
2. National Asthma Education Program (1991) Guidelines for the diagnosis and management of asthma. J Allergy Clin Immunol 88 [Suppl]:425-534
3. Cookson JB (1987) Prevalence rates of asthma in developing countries and their comparison with those of Europe and North America. Chest 91:97S-103S
4. Robin ED (1988) Death from bronchial asthma. Chest 93:614-618
5. Busse WW (1989) The role of inflammation in asthma. J Resp Dis 10:72-80
6. Wenzel SE (1994) Asthma as an inflammatory disease. Ann Allergy 72:261-271
7. Bardana Jr E (1992) What characterizes allergic asthma? Ann Allergy 68:371-373
8. Hahn DL, Beasley JW (1994) Diagnosed and possible undiagnosed asthma: a Wisconsin Research Network (WReN) study. J Fam Pract 38:373-379
9. Burrows B, Martinez F, Halonen M, Barbee RA, Cline MG (1989) Association of asthma with serum IgE levels and skin-test reactivity to allergens. New Engl J Med 320:271-277
10. Hahn DL (1993) Another possible risk factor for airway disease. Chest 104:649
11. Kroegel C, Virchow J-C, Walker C (1993) Asthma. New Engl J Med 328:1639-1640
12. Frigas E, Gleich GJ (1986) The eosinophil and the pathophysiology of asthma. J Allergy Clin Immunol 77:527-537
13. Bivings L (1940) Asthmatic bronchitis following chronic upper respiratory infection. JAMA 115:1434-1436
14. Chobot R, Uvitsky IH, Dundy H (1951) The relationship of the etiologic factors in asthma in infants and children. J Allergy 22:106-110
15. Fox JL (1961) Infectious asthma treated with triacetyloleandomycin. Penn Med J 64:634-635
16. Ogilvie AG (1962) Asthma: a study in prognosis of 1,000 patients. Thorax 17:183-189
17. Stenius-Aarniala B (1987) The role of infection in asthma. Chest 91:130S-136S
18. Hahn DL, Dodge R, Golubjatnikov R (1991) Association of *Chlamydia pneumoniae* (strain TWAR) infection with wheezing, asthmatic bronchitis and adult-onset asthma. JAMA 266:225-230
19. Hahn DL (1994) Acute asthmatic bronchitis: a new twist to an old problem. J Fam Pract 39:431-435
20. Hahn DL, Golubjantnikov R (1994) Asthma and chlamydial infection: a case series. J Fam Pract 38:589-595
21. Peters BS, Thomas B, Marshall B, Weber J, Taylor-Robinson D, Shaw R (1994) The role of *Chlamydia pneumoniae* in acute exacerbations of asthma. Am J Rersp Crit Care Med 149:34/A
22. von Hertzen L, Leinonen M, Koskinen R, Liippo K, Saikku P (1994) Evidence of persistent *Chlamydia pneumoniae* infection in patients with chronic obstructive pulmonary dis-

ease. In: Orfila J, Byrne GI, Chernesky MA, Grayston JT, Jones RB, Ridgeway GL, Saikku P, Schachter J, Stamm WE and Stephens RS (eds) Proceedings of the Eighth International Symposium on Human Chlamydial Infections. Chantilly, France, Società Editrice Esculapio, Bologna, Italy, pp 473-476

23. Allegra L, Blasi F, Centanni S, Cosentini R, Denti F, Raccanelli R, Tarsia P, Valenti V (1994) Acute exacerbations of asthma in adults: role of *Chlamydia pneumoniae* infection. Eur Respir J 7:2165-2168

24. Hahn DL, Golubjatnikov R (1994) Age at asthma diagnosis, skin test positivity and *Chlamydia pneumoniae* seroreactivity (abstract). Am J Respir Crit Care Med 149:913A

25. Saikku P, Leinonen M, Tenkanen L et al (1992) Chronic *Chlamydia pneumoniae* infection as a risk factor for coronary heart disease in the Helsinki Heart Study. Ann Int Med 116:273-278

26. Falck G, Heyman L, Gnarpe J, Gnarpe H (1994) *Chlamydia pneumoniae* (TWAR): a common agent in acute bronchitis. Scand J Infect Dis 26:179-187

27. Kawane H (1993) *Chlamydia pneumoniae*. Thorax 48:871

28. Bone RC (1991) *Chlamydial pneumonia* and asthma: a potentially important relationship. JAMA 266:265

29. Grayston JT (1988) TWAR: A newly discovered *Chlamydia* organism that causes acute respiratory tract infections. Infections in Medicine 5:215-248

30. Pedersen P, Weeke ER (1987) Epidemiology of asthma in Denmark. Chest 91:1075-1145

31. Smith JM, Knowler LA (1965) Epidemiology of asthma and allergic rhinitis. I. In a rural area. II. In a university-centered community. Am Rev Respir Dis 92:16-38

32. Smith JM (1994) Asthma and atopy as diseases of unknown cause. A viral hypothesis possibly explaining the epidemiologic association of the atopic diseases and various forms of asthma. Annals of Allergy 72:156-162

33. Puolakkainen M, Ukkonen P, Saikku P (1989) The seroepidemiology of *Chlamydiae* in Finland over the period 1971 to 1987. Epidem Inf 102:287-295

34. Klaukka T, Peura S, Martikainen J (1991) Why has the utilization of antiasthmatics increased in Finland? J Clin Epidemiol 44:859-863

35. Forsey T, Darougar S, Treharne JD (1986) Prevalence in human beings of antibodies to *Chlamydia* IOL-207, an atypical strain of chlamydia. J Infection 12:145-152

36. Fleming DM, Crombie DL (1987) Prevalence of asthma and hayfever in England and Wales. Br Med J 294:279-283

37. Dodge RR, Burrows B (1980) The prevalence and incidence of asthma and asthma-like symptoms in a general population sample. Am J Resp Dis 122:567-575

38. Burrows B (1987) The natural history of asthma. J Allergy Clin Immunol 80:375S-377S

39. Grayston JT, Kuo CC, Wang SP, Altman J (1986) A new *Chlamydia psittaci* strain, TWAR, isolated in acute respiratory tract infections. NEJM 315:161-168

40. Grayston JT, Aldous M, Easton A et al (1993) Evidence that *Chlamydia pneumoniae* causes pneumonia and bronchitis. J Infect Dis 168:1231-1235

41. Frydén A, Kihlström E, Maller R, Persson K, Romanus V, Anséhn S (1989) A clinical and epidemiological study of "ornithosis" caused by *Chlamydia psittaci* and *Chlamydia pneumoniae* (strain TWAR). Scand J Infect Dis 21:681-691

42. Hammerschlag MR, Chirgwin K, Roblin PM et al (1992) Persistent infection with *Chlamydia pneumoniae* following acute respiratory illness. Clinical Infectious Diseases 14:178-182

43. Emre U, Roblin PM, Gelling M et al (1994) The association of *Chlamydia pneumoniae* infection and reactive airway disease in children. Arch Pediatr Adolesc Med 148:727-732

44. Cunningham A, Johnston S, Julious S, Sillis M, Ward ME (1994) The role of *Chlamydia*

pneumoniae and other pathogens in acute episodes of asthma in children. In: Orfila J, Byrne GI, Chernesky MA, Grayston JT, Jones RB, Ridgeway GL, Saikku P, Schachter J, Stamm WE and Stephens RS (eds) Proceedings of the Eighth International Symposium on Human Chlamydial Infections. Chantilly, France, Società Editrice Esculapio, Bologna, Italy, pp 480-483

45. Marrie TJ (1993) *Chlamydia pneumoniae*. Thorax 48:1-4
46. Hahn DL (1993) Clinical experience with anti-chlamydial therapy for adult-onset asthma. Am Rev Respir Dis 147:297A
47. Hahn DL (1992) *Chlamydia pneumoniae* infection and asthma. Lancet 339:1173-1174
48. Hahn DL, Smith JM (1994) Infection as a cause of asthma. Ann Allergy 73:276
49. Sheth KK, Busse WW (1994) Respiratory tract infections and asthma. In: Gershwin ME and Halpern GM (eds) Bronchial Asthma. Principles of Diagnosis and Treatment. Totowa, New Jersey, Humana Press, pp 481-512
50. Burr ML (1987) Is asthma increasing? J Epidemiol Comm Health 41:185-189

Chapter 10   *Chlamydia pneumoniae* Pneumonia: Radiological Features

FRANCO DENTI, LUIGI ALLEGRA AND FRANCESCO BLASI

Introduction

The most common symptomatic infection sustained by *Chlamydia pneumoniae* is pneumonia [1]. This pathogen is involved in more than 10 % of community-acquired pneumonias with a usually mild to moderate clinical course. However, severe pneumonias are described in patients with underlying diseases [2-4].

Radiographic pattern is estremely variable with a reported high incidence of subsegmental consolidation [5, 6].

Chest x-Ray Description

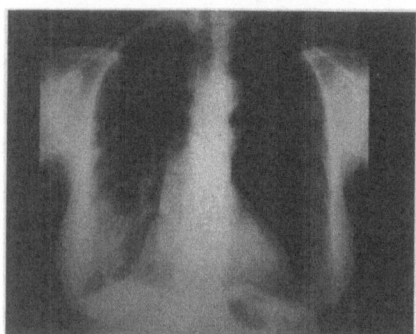 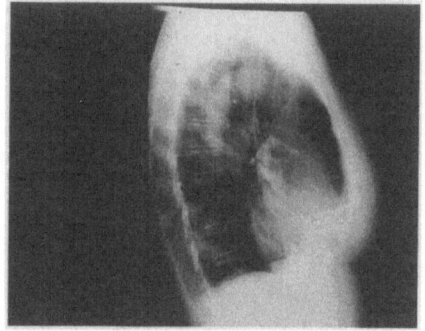

Figs. 1, 2. Posteroanterior (PA) and lateral (L) views of a heterogeneous density pulmonary consolidation in the middle lobe with mild pleural involvement

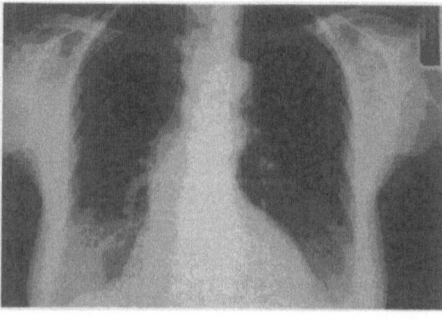

Fig. 3. Less extensive anatomic distribution of the consolidation shown in Fig.1 and complete clearing of the pleural involvement

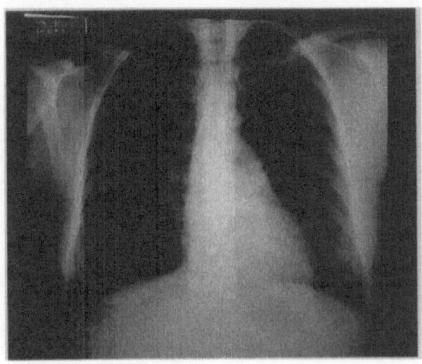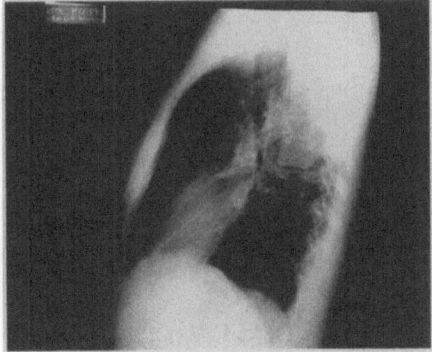

Figs. 4, 5. PA and L views of a ground-glass pattern lingular consolidation

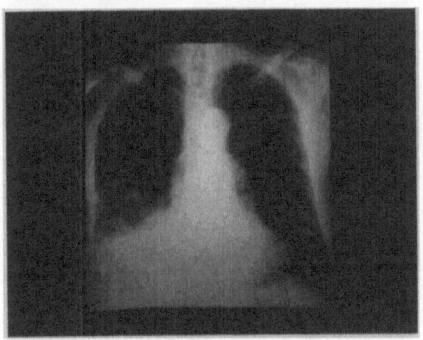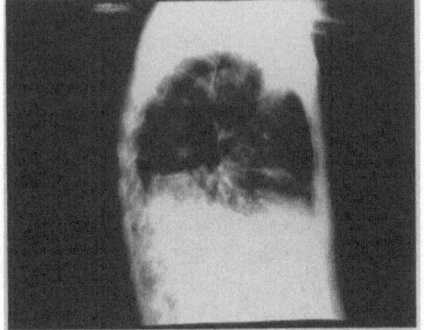

Figs. 6, 7. PA and L projections of a right basilar pleuro-pneumonitis with involvement of the major horizontal right fissure

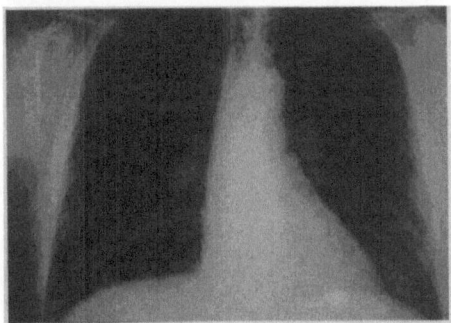

Fig. 8. Initial chest radiograph (PA) of a small poorly defined interstitial right basilar infiltrate

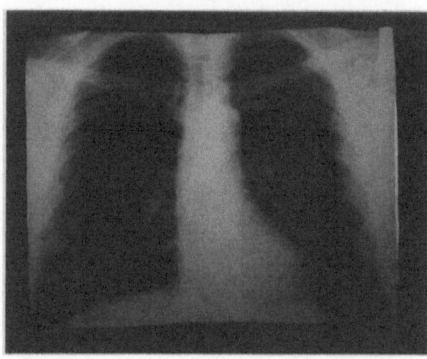
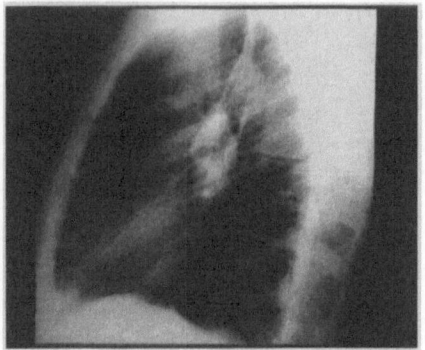

Figs. 9, 10. PA and L views showing complete resolution of the infiltrate described in Fig. 8 following treatment with macrolides

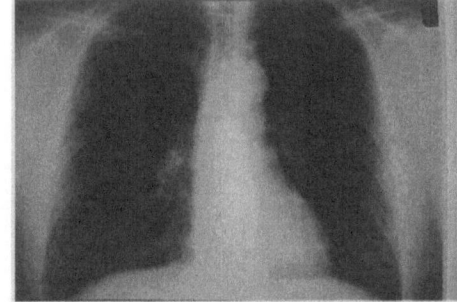

Fig. 11. PA projection of a heterogeneous density right paracardiac infiltrate with ipsilateral hilar adenopathy

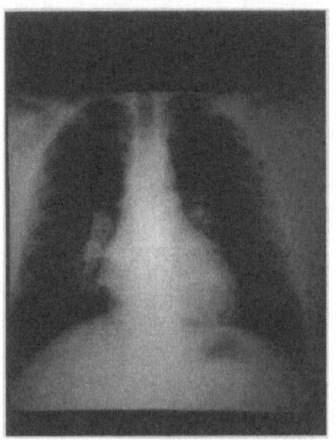
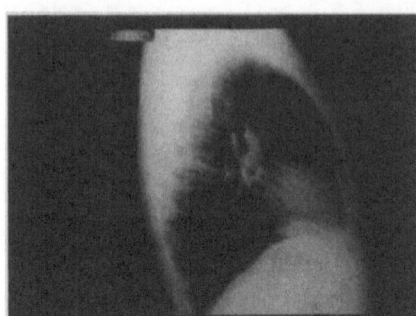

Figs. 12, 13. PA and L views of an interstitial infiltrate involving the apical segment of the right lower lobe

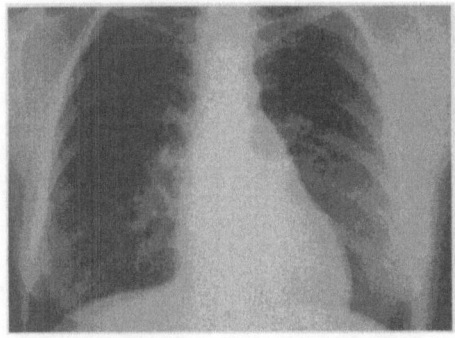

Fig. 14. PA view of a diffuse pulmonary infiltrate of the left upper lobe

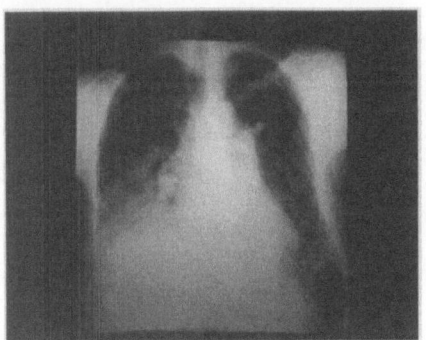
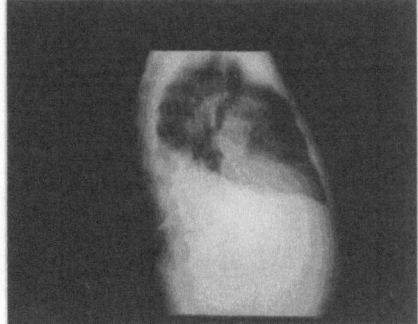

Figs. 15, 16. PA and L views of a large patchy right basilar alveolar consolidation with pleural effusion

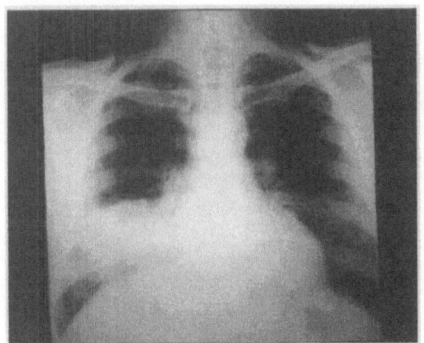
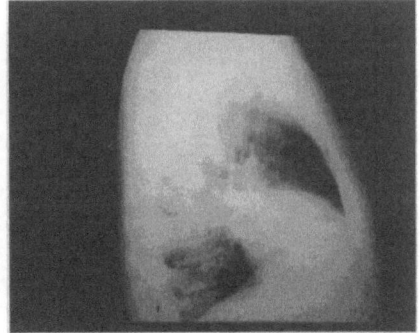

Figs. 17, 18. PA and L views of a pulmonary consolidation of the middle lobe. A smaller contralateral infiltrate is also present

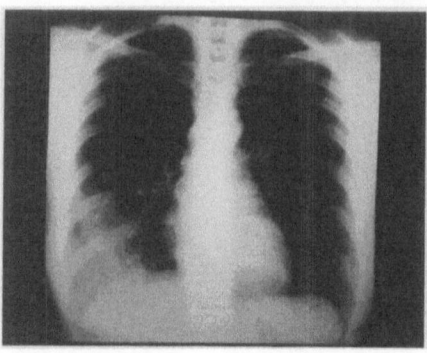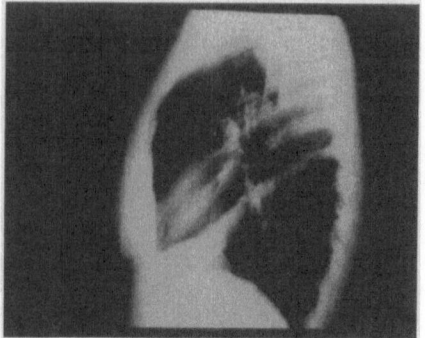

Figs. 19, 20. PA and L views of a right basilar pleuro-pneumonitis with involvement of the major right fissure

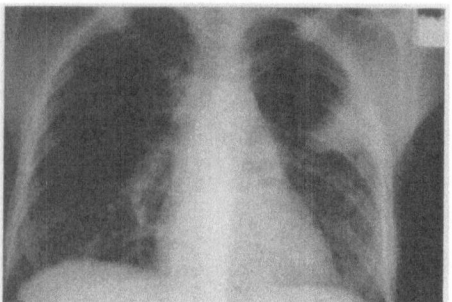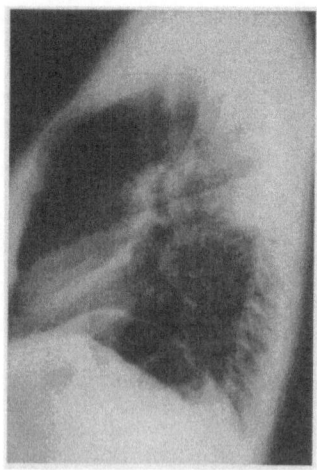

Figs. 21, 22. PA and L views of a small homogenous subsegmental consolidation involving left posterior axillary zone in a young patient with HIV-1 infection

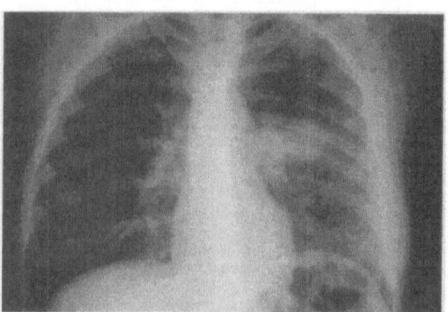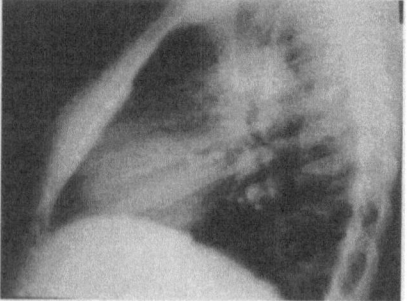

Figs. 23, 24. PA and L views of a small left parahilar homogenous subsegmental infiltrate reaching the ipsilateral hilum in a HIV-1 infected patient

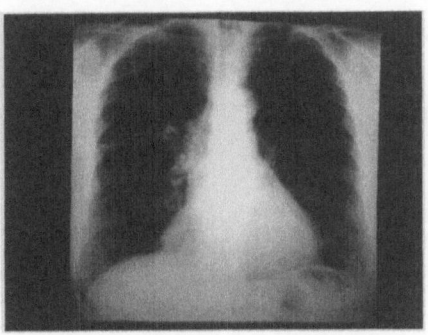 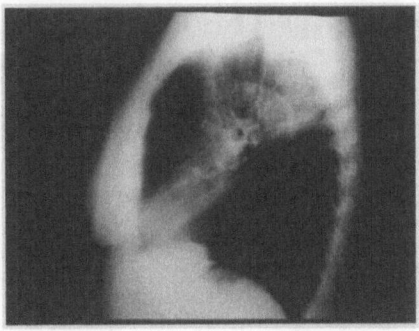

Figs. 25, 26. PA and L views of an interstitial infiltrate involving the upper right lobe

References

1. Thom DH, Grayston JT (1991) Infections with *Chlamydia pneumoniae* strain TWAR. Clin Chest Med 12:245-256
2. Fang GD, Fine M, Orloff J, Arisumi D et al (1990) New and emerging etiologies for community-acquired pneumonia with implications for therapy. Medicine 69:307-316
3. Grayston JT, Diwan VK, Cooney M, Wang SP (1989) Community and hospital-acquired pneumonia associated with *Chlamydia* TWAR infection demonstrated serologically. Arch Intern Med 149:169-173
4. Marrie TJ, Grayston JT, Wang SP, Kuo CC (1987) Pneumonia associated with TWAR strain of *Chlamydia*. Ann Intern Med 106:507-511
5. Marrie TJ, Durant H, Yates L (1989) Community-acquired pneumonia requiring hospitalization: five years prospective study. Reviews of Infectious Diseases 11:586-599
6. Blasi F, Cosentini R, Legnani D, Denti F, Allegra L (1993) Incidence of community-acquired pneumonia caused by *Chlamydia pneumoniae* in Italian patients. Eur J Clin Microbiol Infect Dis 12:696-699

Chapter 11 Perspectives and Perceptions on the Clinical Relevance of *Chlamydia pneumoniae* Infection

Luigi Allegra and Francesco Blasi

Introduction

The contributions present in this book illustrate the importance and the relevance in both respiratory and extrapulmonary diseases of *Chlamydia pneumoniae* infection today. The wealth of knowledge concerning this pathogen has increased dramatically in less than a decade and is analytically represented in the different chapters included in the book.

The microbiological aspects of this third Chlamydia species have now been sufficiently well documented but there are still lines of future research that will have to be pursued. For example, the possible applications of the PCR technique in this field are being currently explored and the use of this test may lead to a fuller understanding of the mechanisms underlying the pathogenesis of chronic infections.

The updating of clinical and epidemiological data present in the book underlines the worldwide diffusion and the wide spectrum of disease presentation of *Chlamydia pneumoniae* infection.

However, many lines of research remain open; in this chapter we will highlight the most interesting ones.

Chlamydia pneumoniae Infection in the Immunocompromised Host

So far only few reports have addressed the clinical importance of *Chlamydia pneumoniae* in the immunocompromised host. Two papers reported evidence of *Chlamydia pneumoniae* infection in HIV-1 positive patients [1,2]. Augenbraun et al. [1] reported an incidence of 10 % of bronchoalveolar lavage specimens positive for *Chlamydia pneumoniae* in HIV patients with unexplained pulmonary processes. Clark et al. [2] described a case of an HIV patient with pneumonia sustained by *Chlamydia pneumoniae*. Moreover it has been recognised that in HIV-1 infected patients *Chlamydia pneumoniae* seroprevalence is higher than in the general population, both in adults and in children [3]. Recently Blasi et al. [4] reported an outbreak of *Chlamydia pneumoniae* infection in an ex-injection-drug users community. A higher *Chlamydia pneumoniae* infection rate in HIV-1 positive subjects may explain the greater morbidity observed in their patients; in fact, more than 76% of HIV-1 positive patients compared to only 38% of HIV-1 negative subjects suffered from acute *Chlamydia pneumoniae* infections. Moreover, most of pneumonias occurred in HIV-1 positive patients and the clinical course of pneumonia was usually more severe than in non-immunocompromised subjects. These data suggest that diagnostic approach to respiratory tract infections in HIV-1 patients should take into account the role of *Chlamydia pneumoniae*.

These reports are consistent with the elegant studies performed by Leinonen and co-workers and here reported in the chapter " Immunology of *Chlamydia pneumoniae* " where the importance of cellular mediated immunity in the response to infection is illustrated.

The role of *Chlamydia pneumoniae* infection in immunocompromised patients seems to be relevant but needs further epidemiological evaluation. However, the most intriguing question is if this intracellular pathogen could affect the natural history of HIV-1 infection. We think that future epidemiological, clinical and laboratory studies will address this interesting topic.

Chlamydia pneumoniae Infection in Chronic Bronchitis and Asthma

Chronic obstructive pulmonary disease (COPD) is still a major cause of morbidity and mortality in many countries. Smoking has been identified as the principal risk factor [5], but only a minority of COPD cases can be explained by smoking [6]. The role of infections in this disease is still controversial. However, some data on the importance of *Chlamydia pneumoniae* infection have been recently published [7,8,9]. Beaty et al. [7] reported an incidence of acute exacerbations of COPD caused by *Chlamydia pneumoniae* of about 4%; these data were confirmed, in a case-control study, by Blasi et al [8] who found an incidence of 5% in a large sample of patients (n=142) with acute exacerbations. They also found a significantly higher seroprevalence for IgG in COPD patients than in controls. This stronger prevalence could indicate the presence of chronic infection by *Chlamydia pneumoniae* , as suggested by the reported increase of specific IgG prevalence and geometric mean titre with age. These data have been confirmed by von Hertzen et al [9] who found high stable IgA serum levels in their COPD patients providing further evidence for an association of *Chlamydia pneumoniae* with COPD.

The possible role of *Chlamydia pneumoniae* in the etiopathogenesis of chronic bronchitis needs to be further evaluated, with a special regard to the possible link between this infection and chronic bronchial inflammation.

A further line of research is the evaluation of the potential role of *Chlamydia pneumoniae* in the pathogenesis of bronchial asthma. Preliminary reports apparently indicate the existence of a link between *Chlamydia pneumoniae* infection and asthmatic exacerbations and suggest a role for this agent in the onset of asthma [10,11]. Hahn et al [10] reported a possible association of *Chlamydia pneumoniae* infection with wheezing and adult-onset asthma. The results of this study showed a dose-response relationship between specific antibody titre level and prevalence of wheeze; moreover, 4 out of 19 patients with acute *Chlamydia pneumoniae* infection subsequently developed asthma, and four others had exacerbation of previously diagnosed asthma. Allegra et al [11] showed that acute exacerbation of asthma was associated with infection in 20% of their patients; interestingly, viruses were involved in about 9% of asthma attacks, while acute infection with intracellular bacteria was detected in 11% of cases. Notably, most of the latter (7/8 cases) were due to *Chlamydia pneumoniae* infection.

The possible link between *Chlamydia pneumoniae* infection and asthma has been highlighted here by Hahn in the chapter " Evidence for *Chlamydia pneumoniae* infection in asthma" , providing a plausible framework for future research into primary causation of asthma.

Chlamydia pneumoniae Infection and Atherosclerosis

Undoubtedly the most sensational progress in our knowledge could derive from the full understanding of the so far only hypothetical association between *Chlamydia pneumoniae* infection and atherosclerosis. The initial intuition regarding this correlation belongs to Saikku [12] who has fully addressed this topic in the chapter on "Chronic infections", written for this book. Very recent data [13] from our Research Group show a possible *Chlamydia pneumoniae* involvement in the etiopathogenesis of aortic aneurysm and additional evidence for an association between this agent and atherosclerosis. In 49% of 37 surgical specimens of aortic aneurysm plaque a nested-polymerase chain reaction for *Chlamydia pneumoniae* DNA detection resulted positive. All patients but one, who resulted seronegative, with PCR-positive plaque showed a *Chlamydia pneumoniae* antibody pattern indicating past or chronic infection. Among patients with PCR-negative plaque, 26% had high *Chlamydia pneumoniae* antibody titre, 32% an antibody pattern indicating past or chronic infection, and 42% were seronegative. Seropositivity for *Chlamydia pneumoniae* was significantly higher in subjects with PCR-positive plaques than in subjects with PCR-negative plaques.

If the relationship between *Chlamydia pneumoniae* chronic infection and atherosclerosis will be proved correct in the future there may be a truly revolutionary impact on the prevention and therapy of atherosclerosis and ischemic heart disease.

References

1. Augenbraun MH, Roblin MR, Chirwing K, Landman D, Hammerschlag MR (1991) Isolation of *Chlamydia pneumoniae* from Lungs of Patients Infected with the Human Immonodeficiency Virus. J Clin Microbiol 29:401-402
2. Clark R, Mushatt D, Fazal B (1991) Case Report: *Chlamydia pneumoniae* Pneumonia in an HIV-Infected Man. Am J Med Sci 302(3):155-156
3. Blasi F, Cosentini R, Clerici Shoeller M, Lupo A, Allegra L (1993) *Chlamydia pneumoniae* seroprevalence in immunocompetent and immunocompromised populations in Milan. Thorax 48:1261-1263.
4. Blasi F, Boschini A, Cosentini R, Legnani D, Smacchia C, Ghira C, Allegra L (1994) Outbreak of *Chlamydia pneumoniae* Infection in Former Injection-Drug Users. Chest 105:812-815

5. Davis RM, Novotny TE (1989) The Epidemiology of Cigarette Smoking and Its Impact on Chronic Obstructive Pulmonary Disease. Am Rev Respir Dis 140:S82-S84
6. Fletcher C, Peto R, Tinker C, Speizer F (1976) The Natural History of Chronic Bronchitis and Emphysema. Oxford, Oxford University Press
7. Beaty CD, Grayston JT, Wang SP, Kuo CC, Reto CS, Martin TR (1991) *Chlamydia pneumoniae*, Strain TWAR, Infection in Patients with Chronic Obstructive Pulmonary Disease. Am Rev Respir Dis 144:1408-1410.
8. Blasi F, Legnani D, Lombardo VM, Negretto GG, Magliano E, Pozzoli R, Chiodo F, Fasoli A , Allegra L (1993) *Chlamydia pneumoniae* Infection in Acute Exacerbations of COPD. Eur Respir J 6:19-22
9. von Hertzen L, Leinonen M, Koskinen R, Liippo K, Saikku P (1994) Evidence of Persistent *Chlamydia pneumoniae* Infection in Patients with Chronic Obstructive Pulmonary Disease. In : Orfila J, Byrne GI et al. (eds), Proceedings of the Eighth International Symposium on Human Chlamydial infection, Chantilly, France, Società Editrice Esculapio, Bologna, Italy. pp 473-476
10. Hahn DL, Dodge RW, Golubjatnikov R (1991) Association of *Chlamydia pneumoniae* (Strain TWAR) Infection with Wheezing, Asthmatic Bronchitis, and Adult-onset Asthma. JAMA 266: 225-230.
11. Allegra L, Blasi F, Centanni S, Cosentini R, Denti F, Raccanelli R, Tarsia P, Valenti V (1994) Acute Exacerbations of Asthma in Adults : Role of *Chlamydia pneumoniae* Infection. Eur Respir J 7:2165-2168
12. Saikku P, Leinonen M, Mattila K, Ekman MR, Nieminen MS, Makela PH, Huttunen JK, Valtonen V (1988) Serological Evidence of an Association of a Novel Chlamydia, TWAR, with Coronary Heart Disease and Acute Myocardial Infarction. Lancet ii: 983-986
13. Blasi F, Denti F, Erba M, Cosentini R, Raccanelli R, Rinaldi A, Fagetti L, Esposito G, Ruberti U, Allegra L Detection of *Chlamydia pneumoniae* in Atherosclerotic Plaques of Aortic Aneurysms. N Engl J Med (submitted)

Subject Index

A

B

C

O

ofloxacin 25, 28, 36

P

penicillin 32, 36
periodicity 18
photon microscopy 4
pneumonia 33, 76
pneumonia outbreaks 16
polymerase chain reaction (PCR) 10, 12, 70, 84
prevalence 33
primary infection 18, 31, 41, 42, 45, 46
proteins 40

R

radiological features 76
reactive airway disease 71
reactive arthritis 56
reinfection 18, 31, 41, 42, 44, 46
replication 3
respiratory tract infections 15, 31, 54, 56
reticulate bodies 5, 10, 12, 39
roxithromycin, 25

S

sarcoidosis 17, 40, 55
seasonal periodicity 18
serologic tests 12
serology 12, 52
seroprevalence 15, 16, 83
sparfloxacin 25, 28
species antigens 6

T

T-cell 42, 43, 45
T-cell mediated immunity 43, 44, 46
taxonomy 3
tetracycline 24, 28, 33, 34, 35, 36